Praise for *The Metabolic Balance Kitchen*

"These recipes can change your life! Jane's insightful knowledge therapy provide the 'ingredients' for successful dieting and overall good health."
Lawrence B. Cohen, MD, gastroenterologist at Cleveland Clinic Canada
and associate professor of medicine at the University of Toronto

"Nutrition is the foundation for optimal health. I believe these recipes
in *The Metabolic Balance Kitchen* can enhance your life!"
Dr. Ira Bernstein

"Jane Durst-Pulkys is an excellent holistic nutritionist and a wellness sage. Her gifts are quite remarkable. With her guidance, individuals can pinpoint and address health issues and know with confidence how to overcome them through great nutrition and Jane's smart recipes. *The Metabolic Balance Kitchen* will be a big hit and helpful to many people!"
Elizabeth Papadopoulos, founder of the Institute of Holistic Nutrition

"This new cookbook, *The Metabolic Balance Kitchen*, will take readers on a journey to a happier, healthier life! Jane Durst-Pulkys is not only a nutritional expert, but she is also highly skilled in understanding cause and effect in the disease process. Her recipes help balance the functions of the organs through diet and nutrition and can create remarkable results."
Dr. Michael Stern, founder of Total Tension Release

"I've been working with Jane on the Metabolic Program and have seen great results. I have lost weight (still a bit more to go), but most of all, I feel happier, more energetic, look healthier, sleep better, my headaches are gone, and I've learned how to eat properly . . . *The Metabolic Balance Kitchen* is packed with all sorts of interesting ways to mix up my meals and make meal prep more exciting!"
Jennifer Sparks, vice president of marketing at AspectHealth

"As a chef, I found it easy to follow the Metabolic Balance program, and I enjoyed the benefits of a restored metabolism, a reduction in inflammation, and weight loss. I lost over 60 pounds! Jane has set you up for success with *The Metabolic Balance Kitchen*, with a wonderful array of tasty recipes and a personal plan for overall vitality. Enjoy your Metabolic Balance journey!"
Pam McDonald, chef, food stylist, and creator of *More Than Food*

"Jane Durst-Pulkys is one of the most talented health practitioners with whom I have had the privilege of working. I am very excited about this new cookbook for health and happiness! People everywhere will love *The Metabolic Balance Kitchen*!"
Raymond Aaron, coauthor of *Chicken Soup for the Canadian Soul*

See testimonials on page 234

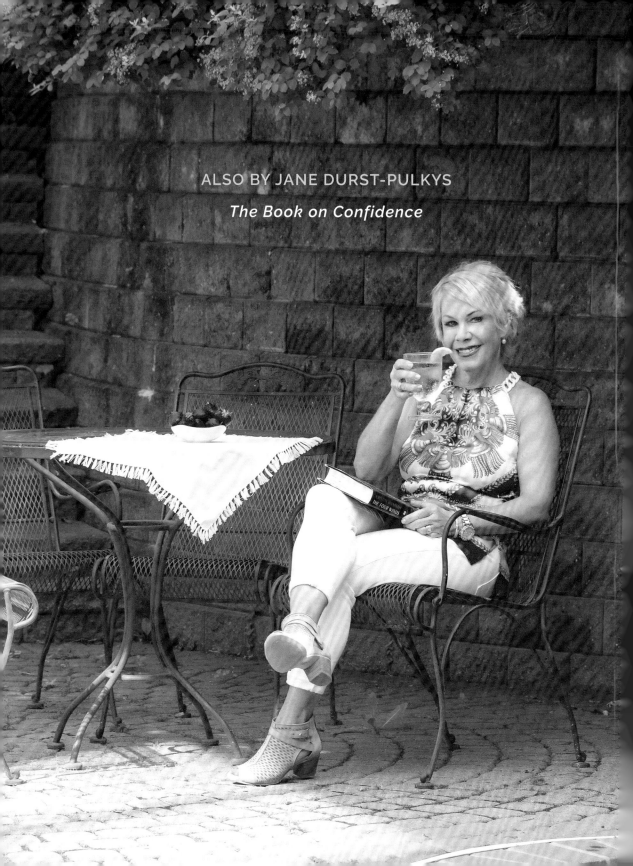

ALSO BY JANE DURST-PULKYS

The Book on Confidence

Deliciously Satisfying Recipes
to Reset Your Metabolism,
Fight Inflammation, and Lose Weight

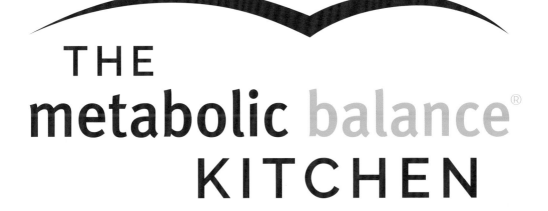

THE
metabolic balance®
KITCHEN

JANE DURST-PULKYS, PhD

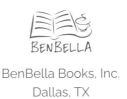

BenBella Books, Inc.
Dallas, TX

BenBella Books, Inc.
10440 N. Central Expressway
Suite 800
Dallas, TX 75231
benbellabooks.com
Send feedback to
feedback@benbellabooks.com

Library of Congress Control Number:
2023024297

ISBN 9781637743843 (paperback)
ISBN 9781637743850 (electronic)

Editing by Claire Schulz
Copyediting by Karen Wise
Proofreading by Lisa Story and Sarah Vostok
Indexing by WordCo Indexing Services, Inc.
Text design and composition by Tara Long
Cover design by Morgan Carr
Printed by KS Printing

Special discounts for bulk sales
are available. Please contact
bulkorders@benbellabooks.com.

This book is dedicated to you, the reader.
As they say in my hot yoga class:
"You're never too old, never too bad,
never too late, never too sick!"
There is always a way to regain and
maintain your health and happiness.

Contents

Introduction

When Joanne first came to my office, I could see right away how unhappy she was with her health. Hitting menopause early had taken its toll, and it seemed like she was constantly full of aches and pains. She didn't sleep well and had no energy. Her joy was gone. She was also heavier than she had ever been, and she didn't know what to eat or what to do. She told me that she had tried all the diet plans out there, lost weight . . . and then put it all right back on. I was her last hope!

As a nutritionist, I had heard versions of this story over and over from women and men searching for an answer to their health woes. Two decades ago (not unlike today) there seemed to be an epidemic of people, young and old, with serious weight issues, searching for strategies or products to lose weight and improve their health. In addition, I had observed that when we feel bad about ourselves, it impacts everything from our mood to our physical functioning. Even looking in the mirror becomes difficult because we don't see the "old me" that we expect. Confidence and self-esteem take a major hit—and we feel like we suffer alone, even though we're far from the only ones who have experienced this.

I wanted to change all that. To help my clients achieve their desired weight and manage their symptoms. To empower, educate, and inspire others and help them look and feel fantastic. It was, and still is, my mission!

However, I spent years of my career trying to help clients like Joanne; like many practitioners, I didn't have the tools yet to help others make real change. But I didn't give up the hunt.

I was searching for a truly scientific program that addressed the real reason that people were having such difficulty losing weight. I knew in my heart that there was something out there.

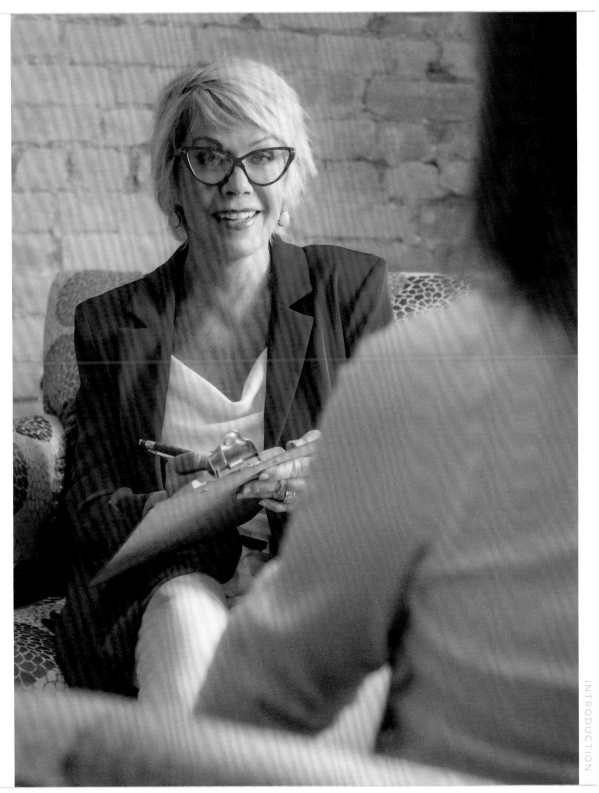

How I Woke Up to the Power of Real Food

From the moment my little fingers could grip the edge of the kitchen table and I could see what Mom was preparing, food simply fascinated me. With 9 children in our family, there was a lot of it around.

Our cleaning lady's husband, Mr. Bray, sold fruits and vegetables to the local produce stores. Every Friday, he pulled up in his huge truck in front of our house and we all ran out to see what he had left over. Mom bought it all: bushel baskets of apples, corn, beans, rhubarb, potatoes, and beets and containers overflowing with strawberries, blueberries, raspberries, and bananas. (I always took 2 bananas and hid them under my bed—they disappeared very quickly, and I wanted to make sure I'd get my share!)

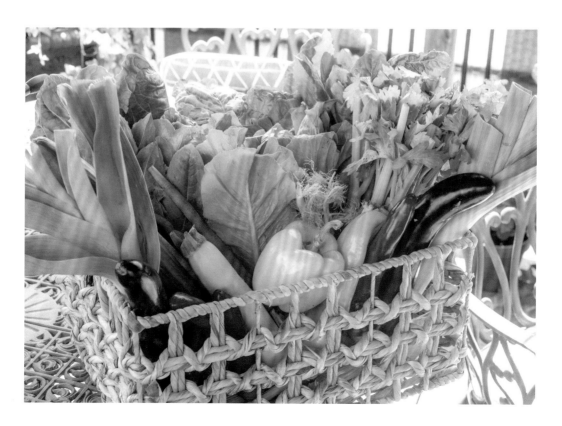

The freshness and flavor of this food made me feel vibrant and alive. All 9 of us kids had huge appetites and a lot of energy. We ran from morning to night with incredible vitality. We stayed on the go and came back to the house only to grab our next meal.

But I don't mean to give you the impression that we subsisted entirely on whole, fresh foods. I was a kid in the 1960s, when households throughout the world—and especially in the United States and Canada—were increasingly embracing convenience foods that supposedly made life easier. Slowly but surely, these processed foods began slipping into our home: powdered milk, Spam, sugary cereals, Velveeta processed cheese that did not even have to be refrigerated, and, of course, sliced white Wonder Bread. My mom bought 25 loaves of Wonder Bread every week, and each night we kids would roll the soft slices into balls and pop them into our mouths.

With these new ingredients in our family's meal rotation, I started packing on the pounds despite my activity level. When I got to high school, I put myself on a strict diet. Each day for lunch I would take 4 pieces of melba toast, 2 slices of cheese, and an apple. Because my diet had so few calories and very little fiber, I constantly felt hungry. At one point, I even became totally constipated for over 2 weeks. It was awful.

In those days, we didn't run to Mom for help. I was an especially independent child and tried to solve my own problems. But finally, I felt so horrible that I confided in her what was going on, and she reluctantly gave me some Ex-Lax to help with my situation. But I knew that using medication was not natural and was not a sustainable solution. It was then that I began to make the connection that what I really needed was to eat more real food!

Suddenly, my interest in health and nutrition intensified and I wanted to know more about how the body worked.

It was then that I began to make the connection that what I really needed was to eat more real food!

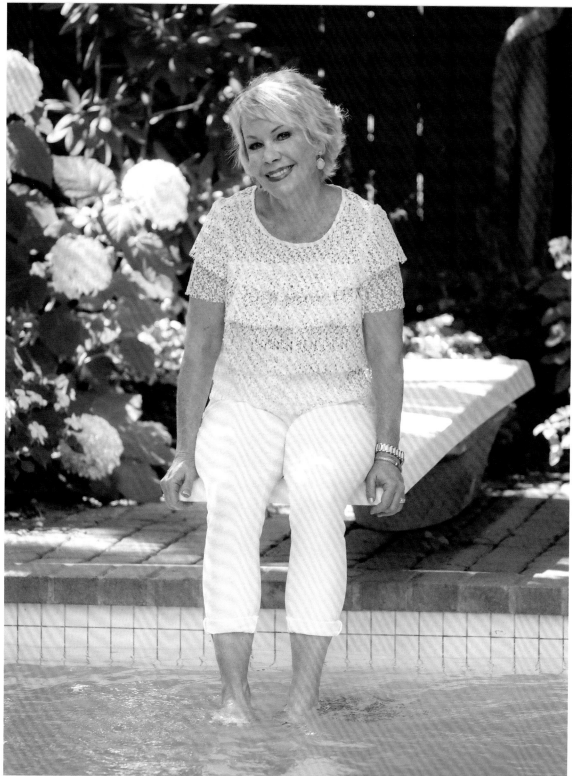

I started out by adding wheat germ to my morning oats and learning how to sprout beans and sunflower seeds, then eventually progressed to planting a vegetable garden, baking my own bread, and making homemade yogurt. I made my own face masks and shampoo, too, using oatmeal and various ingredients from the kitchen. I would store my latest concoction in the refrigerator in a repurposed ReaLemon juice bottle.

One night while my mom was fixing dinner, she opened the bottle and poured my homemade shampoo all over the fish. As I heard my name being emphatically called, I sheepishly walked into the kitchen, thinking I had crossed the line. But what happened next surprised me. Mom looked at me and said, "You need to go to university and study nutrition." My mother saw much more potential in me than she saw in the poor fish that evening, and it ended up in the compost. But for me, that was a pivotal moment in my life and I decided immediately that I would adopt that as my mission.

Four years later, with a bachelor of science degree under my belt, I had my start. My first job was managing a health food store within a large grocery store. I had access to healthy foods, yet my diet was far from perfect. Although I could draw the Krebs cycle (that's one of the steps in our bodies' processing of sugar), name all 22 amino acids, and tell you how much iron was in a serving of Kellogg's Corn Flakes, I didn't yet understand how to eat well. At the university, far from my vegetable garden, I had strayed from homemade yogurt and DIY beauty products and instead joined in with my friends drinking Diet Coke every day and eating Cool Whip and hot bagels. I had also become a marathon runner, and our trainer pushed us to eat carbs, carbs, carbs. To me, that looked like pasta, mass-produced white bread, and anything that would fill me up! As a result, I had terrible allergies and was covered in psoriasis. Clearly, my science studies had not prepared me to understand how to *use* nutrition for optimal health.

> **At last, I was studying nutrition for optimal health, examining natural ways to heal the body.**

That pattern continued even as I got married and started a family. That is, until I decided it was time to follow my earlier passion and go back to school to study holistic nutrition. At last, I was studying nutrition for optimal health, examining natural ways to heal the body. I loved every minute of it and graduated as valedictorian of my class—even while raising three boys! I eliminated the food allergies and hives I had constantly been experiencing, and resolved the autoimmune disease of psoriasis with my new diet. I removed all junk food from my life and my skin and hair began to shine—and my eyes took on a new sparkle.

After graduating, I was pleased to set up my own practice as a nutritionist and I beamed as my first client walked in the door in January 2000. I was excited to share my newfound wealth of information with my clients. Creating individualized meal plans was still a guessing game because I was missing the true science of eliminating inflammation and creating optimal metabolism for clients who want to be healthier and to lose weight. That piece of the puzzle would fit in later, when I learned about Metabolic Balance.

Finding the Answer in Metabolic Balance

One day everything changed—and my career in nutrition was about to take a giant leap forward. A dear friend and colleague told me about a program called Metabolic Balance. With it, she had lost twenty pounds and felt better than she had in years. As it happened, the Metabolic Balance cofounder, Dr. Wolf Funfack, had just come from Germany to Toronto to give a talk that night. I decided I was meant to be there.

When I arrived, the room was packed. I sat down near the back and waited in anticipation for what Dr. Funfack might share. He began to speak, and as I listened carefully my jaw dropped open. What he described was brilliant—true science applied perfectly in a personalized nutritional program designed to optimize the performance of the body, lower inflammation, balance hormones, and reach and maintain a healthy weight (see What Is Metabolic Balance and How Does It Work? on page 18).

The plan was based on healthy food that would make a person feel full and satisfied. And as a practitioner, I was delighted to hear that a client's medications and health concerns could all be factored into their individualized plan.

Magic—that's what it felt like to me. I enrolled in his course and walked out that door with a new purpose. I was excited beyond measure and hit the ground running. I immediately did the program myself and felt amazing.

Cooking Up Health and Happiness

Happiness is the greatest thing that life can offer. Nothing feels better than being happy and healthy. I truly go to bed happy and wake up happy, but it was not always that way. I struggled with confidence when I was a young woman and I've made it my mission to become as happy and confident as possible. I ended up writing a book called *The Book on Confidence*: *Standing Tall on the Inside*. I removed the 7 Deadly Words from my vocabulary: *can't*, *should*, *try*, *must*, *if*, *or*, and *need*. I cleaned up my relationships and decided that my friends had to either help me grow or go. I cultivated my remaining relationships with love and respect, and I am a person who walks around every day feeling grateful for just about everything.

I journal each morning and do a spiritual exercise (meditate, contemplate, or pray) each day. I make sure I have no negative self-talk. I believe in the 80–20 rule, which means that what you do 80 percent of the time matters the most. I have been happily married for over 40 years and I believe the secret is love, respect, and freedom!

I am happy because I choose happiness. There is only one thing in the whole world we can control and that is our attitude. Thank you for being part of my journey, and I wish you well on your journey to health and happiness!

Then, as a Metabolic Balance practitioner, I had access to a professional coach who answered every question and an MD who provided all the medical information I needed. As word spread, my practice began to thrive because of my clients' success.

Metabolic Balance has changed my life. With this program, I've learned about how to eat for enhanced health and energy. I also know how to eat when on vacation so I can travel often without worrying about gaining weight. I know what a "treat meal" is, understand how important the 8 Rules of Metabolic Balance are, and appreciate the many benefits of exercise. And, with this book, I'll share more about all of those topics with you too!

After working with over 1,200 clients, I can truly say this program works beyond anything I have ever seen. The transformation in my clients' health is staggering; I now know what I was missing with Joanne, who was depressed, overweight, and very unhealthy, and I can finally give my clients the tools and strategies to make lasting and effective change. I have seen clients with fatty liver disease who have completely reversed it with a Metabolic Balance program. Others no longer need medications for high blood pressure or other ailments and are able to go off their prescriptions with their doctors' blessings. I've also seen skin cleared, energy returned, and clients looking younger and happier than they ever expected. Some others can finally get pregnant! Each client is different, of course, and not everyone has the same results, but nothing in the world makes me happier than watching my clients finally achieve their goals.

Metabolic Balance is the real deal, and I believe you'll love the taste and the science behind the recipes I'll be sharing with you!

Your Journey Starts Here

Metabolic Balance is represented in over 40 countries, and in this book, I offer you Metabolic Balance–friendly recipes from all over the world, designed to provide many health benefits. Throughout the book, I'll share some of the secrets of the Metabolic Balance program, which can help you reset your metabolism, fight inflammation, and achieve and maintain a healthy body weight.

The aim of this book is to give you an insight into the process of Metabolic Balance by offering you inspiration for the types of healthy and delicious recipes possible with this program. Metabolic Balance is comprised of 3 essential components: unique personalized nutrition plans created for each person; guided support from a trained coach; and fabulous nourishing meals of real, fresh, and nutritious food. While simply enjoying these recipes can give you considerable health benefits, the maximum advantage can truly be achieved when you have your own personalized plan and work with a Metabolic Balance coach. They can guide you through the process (see "What Is Metabolic Balance and How Does It Work?" on page 18). I wish you the best of success with your Metabolic Balance journey.

Throughout the book, I'll share some of the secrets of the Metabolic Balance program, which can help you reset your metabolism, fight inflammation, and achieve and maintain a healthy body weight.

What Is Metabolic Balance and How Does It Work?

Metabolic Balance is a healthy way of life that provides innumerable benefits, including enhanced youthfulness and vitality, and optimal weight and fitness. If you are skeptical, you're not alone. I cannot count how many times clients have walked through the door after trying (and failing) to lose weight, and wondered if Metabolic Balance was just yet another program that would fail. The public has been bombarded with conflicting information for years, and even the experts cannot seem to agree. But science has spoken—and the secret to overall health lies in our hormones!

There are 4 types of hormones that regulate metabolism, and they need to be balanced for optimal health:

1. **Ghrelin** is the hunger hormone that signals for you to eat.

2. **Leptin** is the hormone that signals fullness. It's an appetite suppressant.

3. **Insulin** is the blood sugar balancing hormone. Elevated levels lead to fat storage.

4. **Glucagon** blocks insulin and helps to balance blood sugar.

Various things happen when you have high insulin levels. You are permanently hungry and have food cravings. Fat builds up easily in your body. Your ability to burn fat is blocked. And you age faster. Too much insulin increases the creation of triglycerides and blocks their breakdown. High levels of insulin can also rob you of restful sleep because it impairs your melatonin production, which promotes deep sleep. The Metabolic Balance program

The 8 Rules of Metabolic Balance

1. Eat 3 meals each day (see page 39).

2. After each meal, take a break of 5 to 7 hours (not including sleeping) before your next meal (see page 39).

3. Don't allow a single meal to last longer than 1 hour (see page 39).

4. Always begin each meal with 2 bites of protein (see page 65).

5. Have only 1 complete protein at each meal and eat 3 different protein groups each day (see page 60).

6. If possible, do not eat after 9:00 pm (see page 206).

7. Drink 35 milliliters of water per kilogram of body weight every day, or 1 fluid ounce of water for every 2 pounds of body weight (see page 131).

8. Eat 1 apple each day as part of a meal (see page 34).

Metabolic
Balance is based
on 2 important
assumptions:

Metabolic Balance is based on 2 important assumptions:

1. The human body is capable of producing all the hormones and enzymes it needs for a healthy metabolism.

2. The body has the ability to develop an appetite for foods containing the nutrients that the body needs.

is designed to reset your metabolism and balance hormone levels, particularly insulin, to enable your body to reach its optimal weight. There are 4 phases in the program (which we'll cover shortly) and 8 rules to follow every day—see the boxes on those throughout the book!

We know the Metabolic Balance program works—both from research and from what clients report. Independent studies of the Metabolic Balance nutrition program showed impressive results, including significant improvement in triglyceride levels and cholesterol (both total and LDL and HDL) levels. In one study, 62.5 percent of participants successfully maintained a 5 percent reduction in baseline weight for a period of one year. The level of pain improved significantly across the board. There was also a high level of compliance on the program, which was attributed to having individually designed nutrition plans and personal counseling with a Metabolic Balance coach.

Is the Metabolic Balance Program for Everyone?

Who can participate in the Metabolic Balance program? Pretty much anyone who wants to:

- improve their quality of life
- detox their body
- stay fit into their senior years
- lose weight and keep it off
- increase libido
- decrease blood pressure
- decrease high cholesterol
- manage type 2 diabetes
- decrease pain
- eliminate swelling

- eliminate suffering with fatty liver disease

- improve mental health

- become pregnant*

- have more energy and stop feeling exhausted

- eliminate the feeling of being burned out

- look and feel better

- handle symptoms of menopause

(*The program is not recommended for people who are already pregnant or are nursing.)

How Can You Get a Personalized Metabolic Balance Plan?

The first step to getting your own customized plan is to contact a coach who can help you decide if a Metabolic Balance program is right for you, and will explain the process. This meeting can occur in person or online anywhere in the world. Your coach will want to find out all your health goals and any health challenges you may have. The coach will provide a questionnaire that covers some basic information, like your age, height, desired weight, food preferences, any medications you may be taking, and your waist, hip, and thigh measurements. Your coach will arrange the blood work needed to provide precise information on your health status, organ function, and potential metabolic issues. It also will reveal if you have inflammation and/or if you are at risk of potential problems like heart disease or fatty liver disease. Once those results are ready, the coach will send all your information to MB's headquarters in Germany, where each plan is created.

Your information is analyzed and the results used to determine your individual eating plan to boost your metabolism and create healthy weight loss or weight management. Best of all, this is all accomplished

The CRP Blood Test

Metabolic Balance assesses the degree of inflammation in the body using C-reactive protein (CRP). CRP is a protein made in the liver and is part of the body's immune response. It is released in high levels during infection, injury, or chronic disease. CRP is just 1 of the 36 blood values used by Metabolic Balance to assess a person's health for their plan.

Metabolic Syndrome

Metabolic syndrome, a.k.a. insulin resistance, is a serious health problem around the world. The syndrome is actually a cluster of conditions, including type 2 diabetes, high blood pressure, and abnormal cholesterol or triglyceride levels, that occur together and can increase the risk of stroke and heart disease.

What is causing this global problem of metabolic syndrome? It is our diets. We now have four new food groups: fast, fried, junk, and processed. These foods lack water, fiber, enzymes, and life force. You can recognize many of these foods as they are often beige in color: fries, bagels, muffins, chips, cookies, waffles, and many others. Our digestive systems have a very difficult time with that industrial magic.

These foods are all high in sugar and unhealthy carbohydrates and thus turn into fat. When sugar intake is too high for prolonged periods of time, our body's cells try to protect themselves by taking in more glucose; our insulin receptors, which facilitate this process, become negatively impacted. Ultimately, glucose, the fuel for the brain, drops and energy is depleted. This is how insulin resistance can start.

How do you know if you are at risk for metabolic syndrome? Regardless of how tall you are, or even your build, the size of your waist matters. With a waist size of 35 inches and higher for females or 40 inches and higher for males, you will see the signs of metabolic syndrome.

Why does waist size matter? It all has to do with visceral fat, which is the fat right behind the belly button. This is the fat that, no matter how hard we try, simply won't seem to go away. It often gives the body an apple shape, but even in thin people, visceral fat can be dangerous. This fat wraps around organs (the heart, kidneys, pancreas, and liver) and puts out inflammatory cytokines, which ultimately lead to inflammation and interfere with the hormones that regulate appetite, weight, mood, and brain function. Metabolic Balance targets the visceral fat by providing a diet designed to lower insulin and balance hormones so that an optimal weight can safely and easily be reached.

through the power of real food, with no pills or proprietary powders or shakes. Each food item on your plan will be carefully selected based on its glycemic load, its biological value, and its nutrient content. Low glycemic load foods will be selected on the Metabolic Balance program as they are typically higher in fat, fiber, and/or protein and will make you feel full and satisfied. Foods are chosen with high biological value. This indicates the quality of protein a food contains and how quickly it can be synthesized into protein in the body. Foods are also chosen based on their levels of macronutrients and micronutrients. It is the unique Metabolic Balance analysis that ensures your ideal foods are matched for you. The selected food items are chosen for your specific Metabolic Balance plan and are designed to regulate your metabolism and keep everything in balance for you.

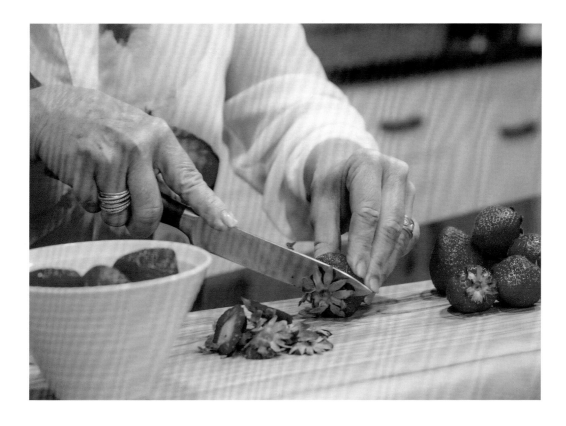

The 4 Phases of Metabolic Balance

Once your MB coach has delivered your personalized plan, you'll begin the 4 phases of the program.

Phase 1: Preparation/Detox

Phase 1 is short and is generally the same for most people. The purpose of phase 1 is to encourage the body, gently and safely, to embrace the new foods and way of eating. It takes place over just 2 days and I always recommend to my clients to find the right time to do this. It's ideal over a weekend or when you can take it easy, stay home, and relax. If you have a coach, then it's essential you follow their advice on what to do on phase 1 as outlined in your plan. In general terms, you start with a gentle digestive cleanse and then eat vegetables for your three meals over the 2 days. During this phase, you cannot have:

- Processed foods

- Caffeinated drinks or soda

- Any type of tea or coffee

- Fruit juice or anything containing sugar or sweeteners

This break from these types of stimulating foods is why some people may not feel so great at the start. The

Resting the Body in Phases 1 and 2

During the first 16 days of your Metabolic Balance program, only minimal exercise is recommended. If you've been exercising hard to lose weight, it can feel odd to stop now—but don't worry, this brief break is worth it. When we rest, the body uses fat as its primary fuel source. At rest, fat constitutes as much as 85 percent of calories burned. That figure shifts to about 70 percent even at an easy walking pace. This is why people can lose between 5 and 20 pounds in the first 16 days even when they are not exercising. Exercise has its place in life—and it's very important—but only after day 16 of resetting your metabolism on the Metabolic Balance program.

body is detoxing, and headaches may occur due to a detox reaction or caffeine withdrawal. My 2 top tips for this phase are first, make sure you drink water regularly throughout your day. A general guide you could use to calculate this is ½ fluid ounce per pound of body weight. So, a 150-pound person would want to drink a minimum of 75 ounces of water (about nine 8-ounce glasses). And next, remember this phase is only for 2 days. You can do this—it's so worth it!

Phase 2: Strict Conversion

The aim of the second phase of the program is to take in optimal nutrition to harmonize your metabolism so you can achieve your desired weight. This phase lasts for at least 16 days, or until you reach your goal. During phase 2, you will need to carefully follow the 8 Rules of Metabolic Balance and closely stick to eating only those foods listed on your personalized food list. This means that the foods people eat during this phase are different for everyone. Believe me, no two plans are exactly alike.

For some people, phase 2 can have two parts. This happens if it takes an individual longer than 16 days to reach their health goals. If so, they'll simply go into an extended phase 2.

During the first 16 days

During the Strict Conversion phase, you eat exactly from your plan. If you are using this book for recipes, remember that all the recipes can be adapted to match the foods on your personalized list. If you are using these recipes without an individualized Metabolic Balance plan, most ingredients are considered core foods, so they will be a great place to start. In addition, if there is a recipe that you like, remember you can always substitute a different protein, like using chicken instead of beef.

Note: No added oils should be used for the first 16 days of phase 2. Cook only with water or veggie broth.

The aim of the second phase of the program is to take in optimal nutrition to harmonize your metabolism so you can achieve your desired weight.

Reducing your fat intake for this short period can support insulin sensitivity. When insulin levels are more balanced in the body, it is easier to lose weight.

In the first 16 days, it is not uncommon to lose between 5 and 20 pounds. Margaret, a 73-year-old client of mine, lost 21 pounds in the first 16 days. By the time most people hit day 16, they feel great and they come to love the Metabolic Balance food list. They report that some foods like sugary desserts and fast foods just don't have the same appeal.

Day 17 and beyond

If you have not reached your goal weight by day 16, you will simply continue to stay in phase 2 until your goal weight is achieved. Folks who have reached their goal weight will move on to phase 3.

However, whether you're staying on phase 2 or moving on to phase 3, on day 17, we typically want everyone to include oil in their cooking, such as coconut oil, ghee, or olive oil.

Whether you are at your goal weight or need to lose some more weight, there are additional changes that can occur, based on your coach's recommendations, like:

• introducing some daily movement or exercise

• introducing a weekly "treat meal"

Phase 3: Relaxed Conversion Phase

By the time you reach phase 3, you have reset your metabolism, decreased inflammation in your body, and achieved your ideal weight! This is when you enter phase 3 to further stabilize your metabolism.

In phase 3, depending on their goals, my clients have dropped anywhere between 5 and 100 pounds, which makes them (and me) feel thrilled. By this time, most people will be feeling renewed, and they often comment

Foods on a Metabolic Balance plan are rich in minerals, fiber, protein, essential fatty acids, and antioxidants. These foods are easily accessible and taste great! Look for boxes throughout this cookbook to learn more about the properties of specific ingredients.

that everything is simply working better. My clients' faces always change at this point, due to the detoxification and their increased water intake. They look and feel younger! Often, they cannot believe the difference in their bodies and are amazed that they have arrived here. Lots of aches and pains have generally disappeared, and often their doctors marvel at the results of their blood work.

Phase 3 is when you tune in more closely to your body's own inner signals. You can experiment with eating increased portion sizes as you need to and add in additional foods, depending on the season and what's fresh in your local food stores.

It is best to remain on phase 3 for at least 2 weeks before transitioning to phase 4, or maintenance.

Phase 4: Maintenance Phase

It is best to remain on phase 3 for at least 2 weeks before transitioning to phase 4, or maintenance. The goal is to maintain your new state of health by following the 8 rules most of the time and continuing to exercise regularly. This keeps your metabolism stable and working optimally. Phase 4 becomes your new, natural lifestyle.

In this phase, you no longer need to weigh your food as you will have now learned the right portion size for you. Most people typically still have their favorite MB breakfasts and lunches (because they love them!), but then

Treat Meal

Metabolic Balance is about balance, balance in your meal plans and balance in life. This is why, once a week, everyone is encouraged to have anything they want for 1 meal. This is not cheating—this is balance!

Treat meals are typically introduced 2 to 4 weeks after starting phase 2 and are about relaxing and enjoying any regular meal once a week. This could be a breakfast, a lunch, or a dinner, but remember the other 2 meals of the day need to be your MB meals. It's often interesting what people choose for their treat meals, as their new balanced metabolism means they may have a greater sensitivity to salt and sugar, so what they previously thought of as a treat no longer has the same appeal.

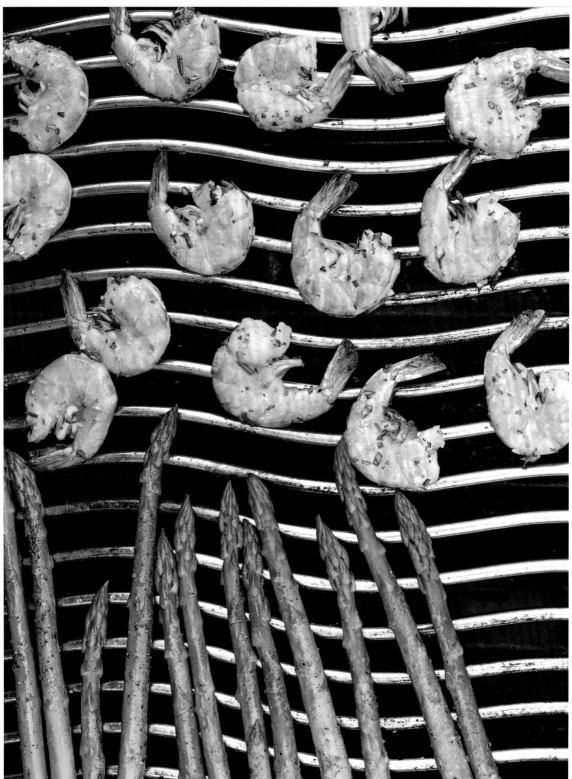

may enjoy more varied healthy dinners. If needed, you can go back to focusing on your ideal food and portion sizes. Most people at this point seem to never want to go back to their old eating habits as they simply feel better eating the Metabolic Balance way. I know for myself, wherever I travel, I am always looking for healthy foods.

It's also great to check in with your coach at regular intervals in order to support your weight loss and healthy lifestyle. The coaching program in Metabolic Balance is one is the keys to success and provides an incredible support system.

Adjusting the Recipes for Your Personalized Metabolic Balance Plan

Throughout this book, I offer recipes with foods often seen on Metabolic Balance food lists, with the quantities in each recipe based on an average calculation. Generally, if you follow the recipes provided—along with the 8 Rules of Metabolic Balance—you will lose weight and decrease inflammation because your body chemistry will change by eating in a more balanced way. Your metabolism will increase and hormones will become more stable as you lose weight. If you are

The Difference a Coach Can Make

I've shared as much as I can so you can get started transforming your health with Metabolic Balance. What I can't fully share is the difference that having a coach can make. Some people think it's their fault if they can't lose weight or stick to healthy lifestyle changes. People also tend to think they should be able to work out all the details by themselves. Scientific evidence and my years of experience have shown that major health shifts are truly successful when people have guided support. A Metabolic Balance coach can provide the skills and knowledge to personalize the program to work best for each individual. Having that guidance allows people to achieve the results they deserve for a healthy and happy future.

Make It a Meal

Most Metabolic Balance dishes (and most of the recipes in this book!) can be accompanied with ½ slice rye bread or 1 rye cracker and a serving of fruit. With many recipes, I've given you a suggestion for some sides. If the recipe does not include veggies, you can add a side salad with vinegar and oil. However, when eating yogurt or oatmeal, rye bread (or rye cracker) is not allowed.

following the Metabolic Balance program with a coach, you will receive your own personalized food plan, including the weight of each food item. It is important for those following their specific plan to use the foods and amounts personally calculated for them, as it varies from person to person. This may alter the recipes slightly, but substitutes can easily be made.

If you don't have a personalized plan, these recipes will give you a good start. The full Metabolic Balance program is designed to help you fight inflammation, reset your metabolism, achieve a healthier weight, and enjoy increased energy and vitality.

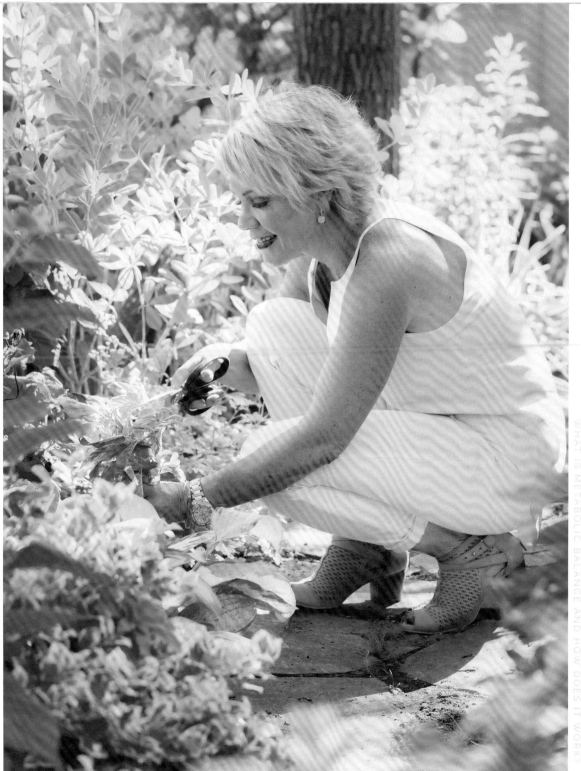

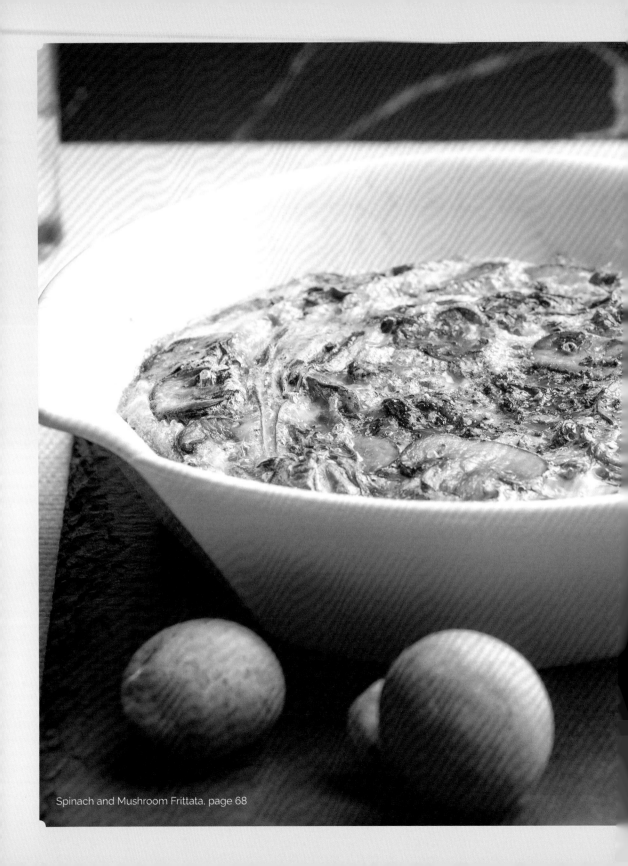

Spinach and Mushroom Frittata. page 68

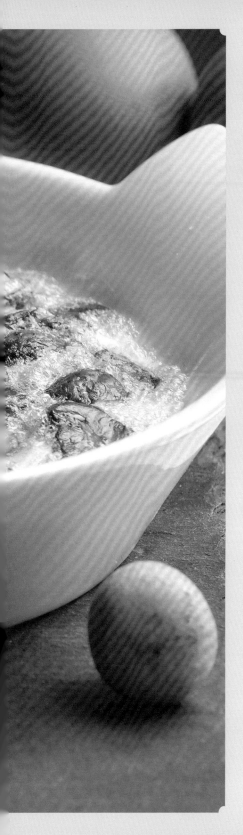

breakfasts

Most of us have heard the saying that breakfast is the most important meal of the day—but it is also my favorite! I can't wait to jump out of bed and decide what I am going to eat each day. It is so important to make time for breakfast as it sets the stage for healthy eating throughout the day. Eating breakfast allows your blood sugar levels to rise at a steady pace throughout the morning. Many people who skip breakfast will tend to overeat later in the day as their blood sugar levels become imbalanced. Eating breakfast the Metabolic Balance way means getting the perfect balance of carbs, proteins, and fats, which helps increase your overall energy throughout the day. My favorites are Apple Oat Delight, Mandelade with Chopped Fruit, and Exceptional Everyday Breakfast Bowl. And for convenience, my Favorite Strawberry Shake is a must!

apple oat delight

This warm, filling breakfast will keep you going until lunch thanks to the substantial helping of fiber from the oats. The aromatic cinnamon reminds me of homemade apple crisp.

Makes 1 serving

¾ cup | 180 mL whole, soy, or goat's milk

1 medium tart apple, cored and finely chopped

½ cup | 50 g rolled oats

2 tsp ground cinnamon

Preheat the oven to 350°F | 175°C.

Mix all the ingredients together in a small baking dish.

Bake for 35 minutes, or until the liquid has been absorbed and the oats are lightly browned. Enjoy warm.

The 8 Rules of Metabolic Balance: #8

Eat 1 apple a day as part of a meal

There is a popular old proverb: "An apple a day keeps the doctor away." It makes sense! No other fruit contains as many vitamins and minerals as the apple. Apples also lower both cholesterol and uric acid, and are rich in pectin and cellulose to provide the body with valuable fiber. This fiber can help with the efficient excretion of harmful metabolic waste products. Old apple varieties like McIntosh, Granny Smith, and Royal Gala are especially rich in polyphenols, which can counteract the effects of free radicals in the body.

See pages 39, 60, 65, 131, and 206 for the other Rules of Metabolic Balance!

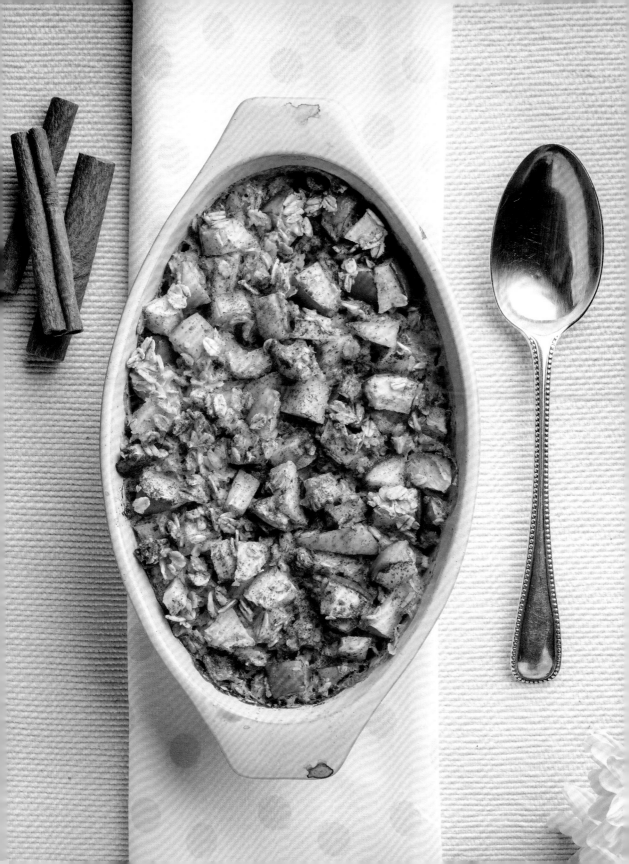

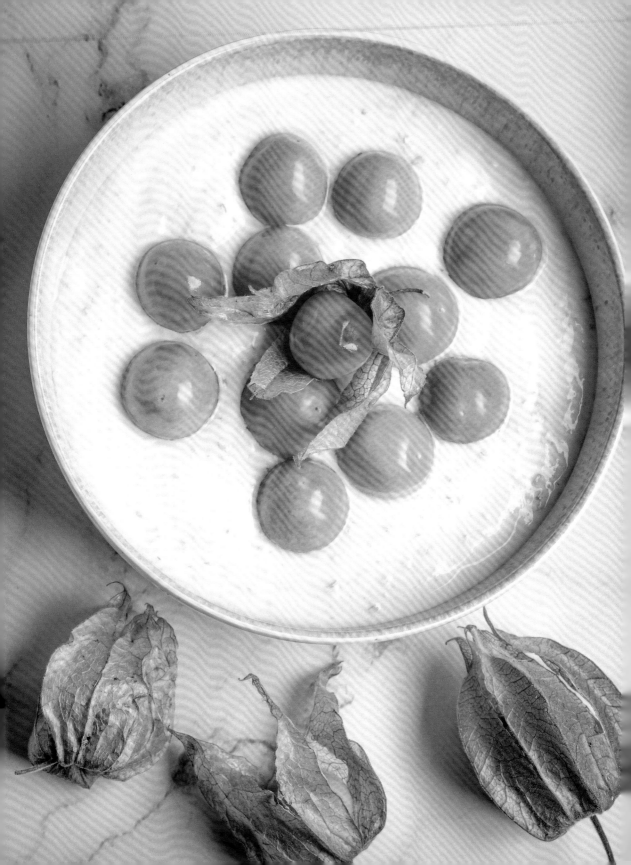

exceptional everyday breakfast bowl

So many of us have busy lifestyles and need something quick but substantial in the morning. This breakfast is my go-to when time is limited and I have an active day ahead. And for me, that's most days, so I make this bowl often!

Health-wise, flax elevates the familiar fruit and yogurt combo from everyday to exceptional: these little seeds are rich in omega-3 fatty acids, which can help lower cholesterol and reduce inflammation. Not to mention, the fiber from the ground flax will help you feel fuller longer.

Makes 1 serving

¾ cup | 170 g
whole-milk yogurt

1 cup | 100 g
gooseberries,
blueberries, raspberries,
or sliced strawberries

2 tbsp | 16 g
ground flaxseeds

½ tsp ground cinnamon

1 tbsp | 15 mL flaxseed oil

1 tbsp | 15 mL water

Eat two bites of the yogurt first to get your protein.

Mix all the ingredients together in a bowl.

Probiotic-Friendly Foods

Probiotics promote the growth of friendly bacteria in the digestive tract. Probiotic-friendly foods include yogurt, sauerkraut, and fermented veggies, which are on most Metabolic Balance plans.

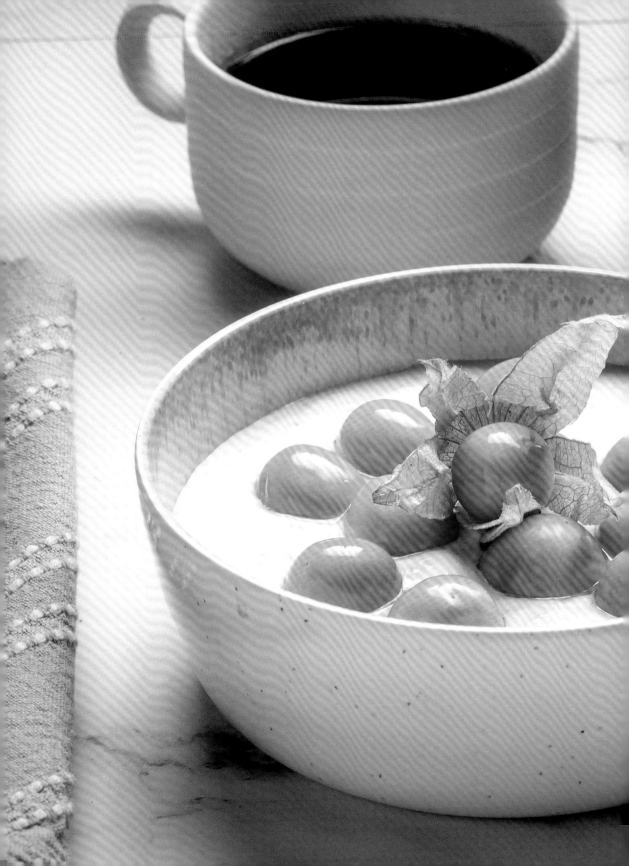

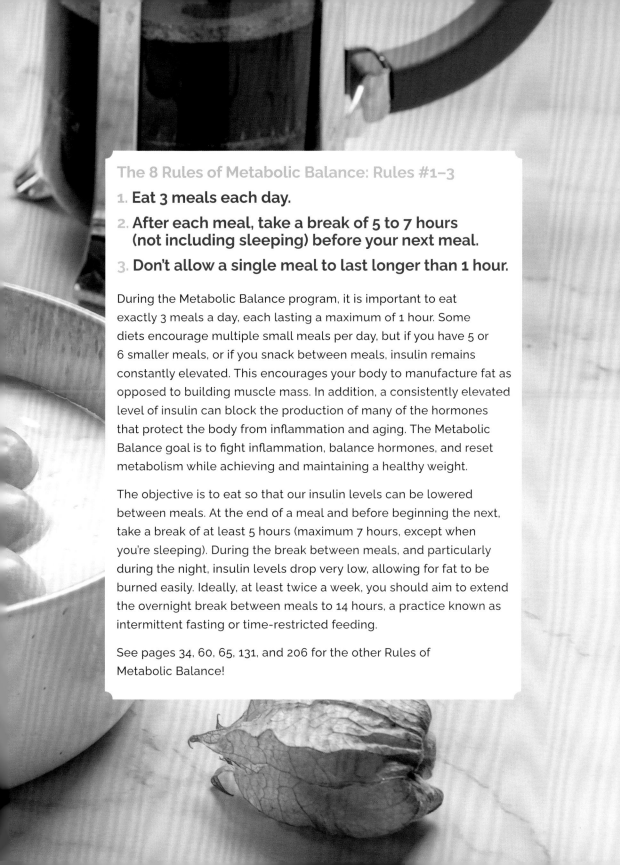

The 8 Rules of Metabolic Balance: Rules #1–3

1. **Eat 3 meals each day.**
2. **After each meal, take a break of 5 to 7 hours (not including sleeping) before your next meal.**
3. **Don't allow a single meal to last longer than 1 hour.**

During the Metabolic Balance program, it is important to eat exactly 3 meals a day, each lasting a maximum of 1 hour. Some diets encourage multiple small meals per day, but if you have 5 or 6 smaller meals, or if you snack between meals, insulin remains constantly elevated. This encourages your body to manufacture fat as opposed to building muscle mass. In addition, a consistently elevated level of insulin can block the production of many of the hormones that protect the body from inflammation and aging. The Metabolic Balance goal is to fight inflammation, balance hormones, and reset metabolism while achieving and maintaining a healthy weight.

The objective is to eat so that our insulin levels can be lowered between meals. At the end of a meal and before beginning the next, take a break of at least 5 hours (maximum 7 hours, except when you're sleeping). During the break between meals, and particularly during the night, insulin levels drop very low, allowing for fat to be burned easily. Ideally, at least twice a week, you should aim to extend the overnight break between meals to 14 hours, a practice known as intermittent fasting or time-restricted feeding.

See pages 34, 60, 65, 131, and 206 for the other Rules of Metabolic Balance!

mango **tea shake**

This is a portable breakfast that satisfies. You'll love the subtle complexity of the tea, the sweet mangoes, and the anti-inflammatory benefit of ginger, which also aids in digestion. Thick and delicious without empty calories, this shake keeps your energy up for a busy day without the mid-morning slump.

Makes 1 serving

¾ cup | 170 g plain whole milk yogurt

1 tsp white tea leaves

¼ cup | 60 mL hot water

1 cup | 145 g cubed mango (fresh or thawed frozen) or strawberries

1 (1-in | 2.5-cm) piece fresh ginger, peeled and thinly sliced

1 lemon balm leaf (optional)

Eat two bites of the yogurt first to get your protein. Combine the tea leaves and hot water in a bowl and let steep, then set aside to cool.

Strain out the tea leaves and pour the tea into a blender. Add the mango, ginger, and yogurt and puree.

Spoon into a large glass and garnish with the lemon balm, if using.

TIP: For the tea preparation, it may be easiest to just brew a bag of tea in a full mug and use ¼ cup | 60 mL for the shake.

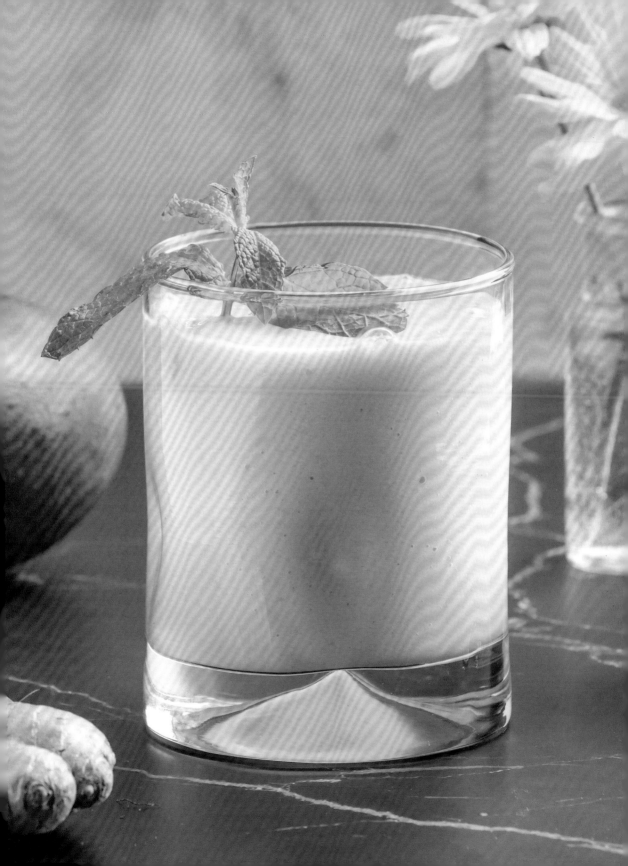

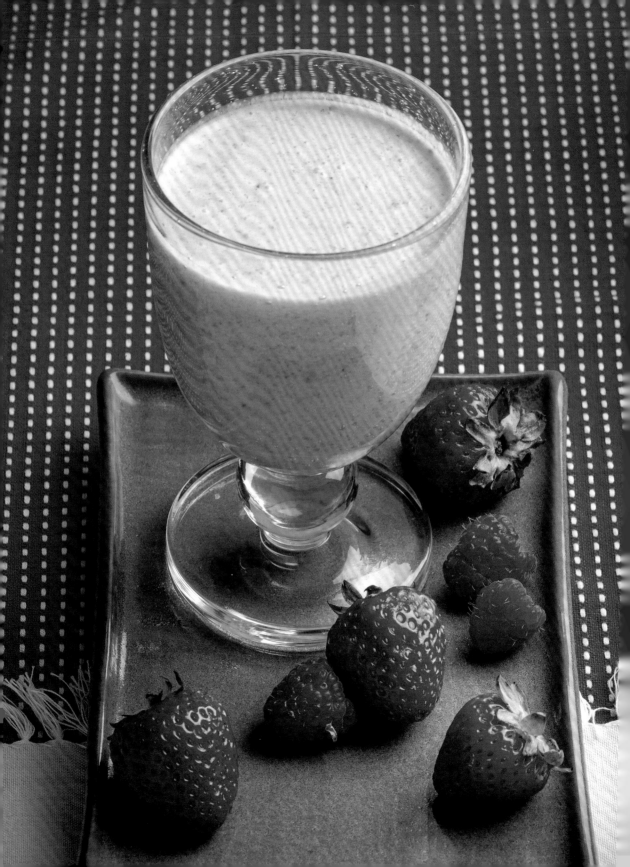

favorite strawberry shake

As a busy nutritionist, I used to rush between meetings with clients, and I found this "sippable" breakfast to be car-friendly! It also packs a huge nutritional punch thanks to the protein in the yogurt, the vitamins in the fruit, and the fiber and omega-3 fatty acids in the flax. The cinnamon is entirely optional, but you may enjoy it; the spice makes food taste sweeter without needing to add sugar. And cinnamon is great for helping reduce triglyceride and cholesterol levels, both of which are risk factors for heart disease. Cinnamon has also been shown to reduce blood pressure when consumed consistently for at least 8 weeks.

Makes 1 serving

¾ cup | 170 g
whole-milk yogurt

1 cup | 100 g strawberries
or other favorite berries

2 tbsp | 16 g
ground flaxseeds

2 tbsp | 30 mL flaxseed oil

Pinch ground cinnamon
(optional)

Eat two bites of the yogurt before blending to ensure you eat your protein first (see box).

Combine the remaining yogurt, the strawberries, flaxseeds, and flaxseed oil in a blender and puree until smooth. If you like, sprinkle on a bit of cinnamon for flavor and a nutritional boost.

Can I have a shake or smoothie while following the Metabolic Balance way of eating?

The answer is yes—as long as you eat two bites of the plain unsweetened yogurt (the protein) before you put it into the blender with the fruit and other ingredients. In the Metabolic Balance program, you must begin each meal with two bites of protein. (Normally, when you have a shake, that cannot happen as the protein-rich yogurt is already blended.) Note that commercial protein powders are not part of the Metabolic Balance program.

toasty seed mix
with onion and tomato

This dish makes a delicious start to the day. The onion and tomato are soft and the seeds add just the right amount of texture. This recipe warms you up from the inside.

Makes 1 serving

2 tbsp | 20 g
pumpkin seeds

2 tbsp | 20 g
sunflower seeds

1 small tomato, diced

½ onion, diced

Salt and black pepper

Put the pumpkin and sunflower seeds in a small bowl and cover with cool water. Cover the bowl and let the seeds soak overnight on the counter.

In the morning, preheat the oven to 350°F | 175°C.

Drain the seeds and rinse well. Mix the seeds, tomato, and onion together in a small baking dish and season with salt and pepper to taste.

Bake for 8 minutes, or until the tomato and onion have softened and the dish is heated through. Enjoy warm.

About the Ingredient: Pumpkin Seeds

Pumpkin seeds can be mixed with almonds as a breakfast meal to create a complete protein. They are loaded with B vitamins, which stress depletes. They also contain hormone-building elements and tryptophan, which helps the body make serotonin and melatonin. Serotonin regulates appetite, mood, emotions, sleep, and even pain. It is the precursor for melatonin, which helps regulate sleep-wake cycles.

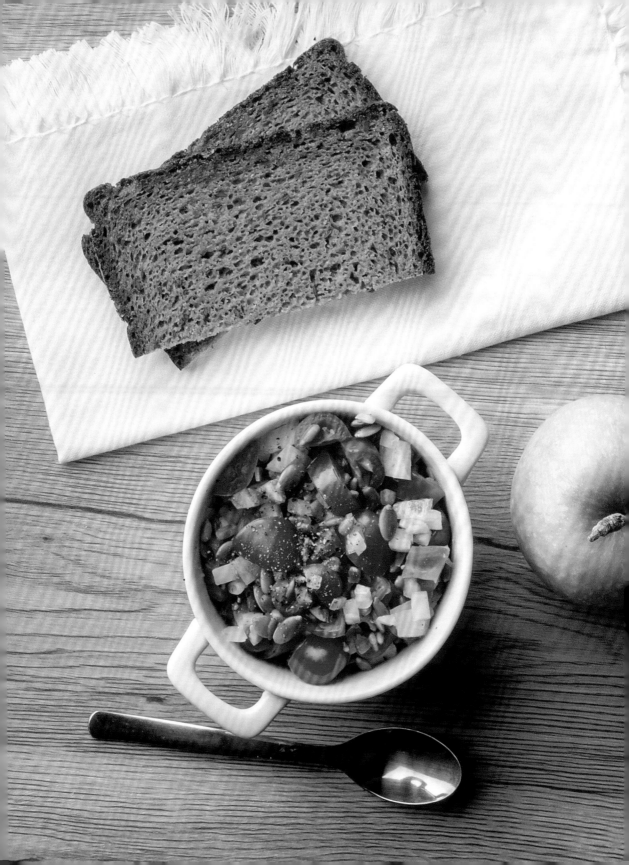

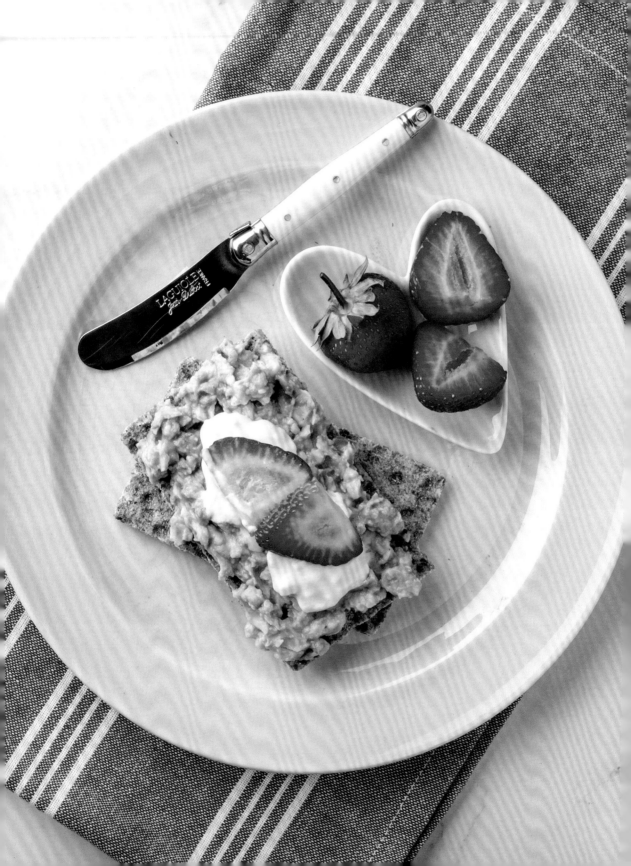

avocado smash
with rye crackers

Eating very colorful foods is a fun way to brighten your day and enhance your health. Crunchy rye crackers make a satisfying base for smooth avocado and cottage cheese. Topped with tangy-sweet strawberries and a drizzle of balsamic vinegar, this dish feels a little fancy but comes together in just minutes.

Makes 1 serving

½ small avocado

1 tsp | 5 mL
fresh lemon juice

2 rye crackers
(such as Wasa or Ryvita)

¼ cup | 60 g full-fat
cottage cheese

4 strawberries,
sliced lengthwise

Balsamic vinegar,
for drizzling

Mash the avocado in a bowl with the lemon juice. Spread the avocado mash on the crackers. Top with the cottage cheese and strawberry slices, then drizzle with balsamic vinegar.

Love Real Food

Ever wonder why we sometimes find ourselves eating the whole basket of white bread at a restaurant? It is because there is nothing in it to make us feel full. With real foods like strawberries and broccoli, we tend not to overeat as they contain juice and fiber, which makes us feel satiated.

However, 100 percent rye bread is added to everyone's Metabolic Balance plan, as it will metabolize slowly and help you feel full longer.

butternut squash and feta spread with rye crackers

Most winter squash—like butternut, acorn, and Hubbard—are loaded with vitamin A, which is an antioxidant. This spread is sweet, savory, creamy, and bursting with flavor.

Makes 1 serving

½ cup | 100 g
cubed butternut squash

2 tsp | 10 mL coconut oil

¼ cup | 40 g
crumbled feta cheese

Salt and black pepper

Pinch fresh thyme leaves
(optional)

2 rye crackers
(such as Wasa or Ryvita)

Preheat the oven to 450°F | 230°C.

In a small baking pan, toss the cubed squash with the coconut oil. Roast for 30 minutes, or until the squash is soft.

Transfer the squash to a bowl and mash with a fork. Stir in the feta cheese and season with salt and pepper to taste. Top with a pinch of thyme, if desired.

Spread on the crackers.

TIP: Cutting up a raw squash can be challenging. A long time ago, I realized if I put a whole squash in a 350°F | 175°C oven for 2 hours, it would slice easily after baking. In this case, you would use 1 cup | 200 g cooked squash and have more left over for soups and other dishes.

About the Ingredient: Coconut Oil

After 16 days on the Metabolic Balance program, clients are asked to eat a total of 3 tablespoons of oil a day (including any oil cooked in a recipe). While a variety of oils are allowed (including coconut oil, ghee, and olive oil), not all oils are created equal! I prefer coconut oil because it is very low in linoleic acid, which the latest research shows is associated with inflammation, heart disease, and other health issues.

When selecting oils, it is important to realize that the vast majority of oils in the grocery store are not pure. Approximately 90 percent of oils (including those labeled as avocado oil and olive oil) are actually adulterated with cheap, oxidized omega-6 vegetable oils, which are harmful to health. When possible, it's best to select coconut oil, ghee, or high-quality olive oil. Whatever oil you're using, always go for the best as good oils can support the cardiovascular system, skin, joints, and hormonal balance.

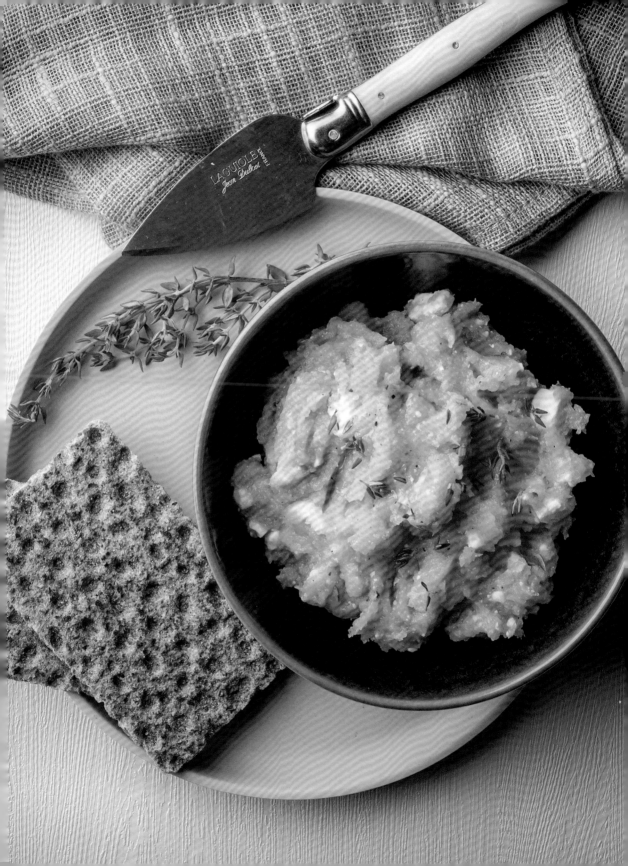

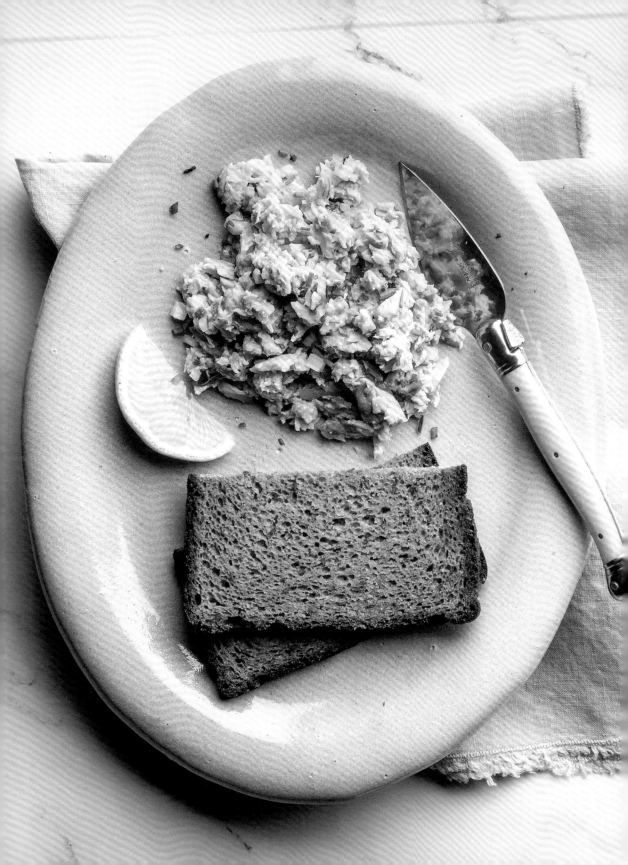

lovely fish breakfast pâté

When it's freezing cold outside in the morning and I want to feel warm and cozy before heading out, I prepare this breakfast. This is an awesome way to enjoy fish in the morning. Made with fresh avocado, chives, and red onion, it wakes up your taste buds.

Makes 1 serving

3½ oz | 100 g salmon, trout, or other firm-textured fish

½ small avocado

2 tsp | 10 mL melted ghee

Dash apple cider vinegar

1 small garlic clove, minced

Salt and black pepper

1 chive, finely chopped (optional)

¼ red onion, finely diced (optional)

2 rye crackers (such as Wasa or Ryvita) or 1 slice rye bread

In a small saucepan, bring about 2 cups of lightly salted water to a boil. Reduce the heat so the water is barely simmering. Gently lower the fish into the water and poach till just cooked through, about 6 minutes. Using tongs or a slotted spoon, transfer the fish to a paper towel to drain and cool slightly. Gently pull the cooled fish apart with a fork.

In a food processor, combine the fish, avocado, melted ghee, vinegar, and garlic and pulse until everything is well combined and the pâté reaches your desired texture. Season with salt and pepper to taste.

Transfer the fish mixture to a small bowl and fold in the chive and/or onion, if using. Cover and chill in the refrigerator for at least 30 minutes, then serve with the crackers or bread.

veggie egg muffins

Eggs are one of the highest-quality sources of protein. They are also an excellent source of the B vitamin choline, which is a key nutrient for brain function and health. Egg muffins are also an excellent breakfast to take with you on the go. Here the muffins are filled with spinach, tomato, onion, and bell pepper, but you can get creative and add any vegetables you like—or whatever vegetables you might have in the refrigerator.

**Makes 1 serving
(3 muffins)**

2 large eggs

2 tsp | 10 mL olive oil

1 small handful
baby spinach

1 small Roma tomato,
diced

1 green onion,
finely chopped

¼ red bell pepper (or any color), cut into small dice

1 small garlic clove,
minced

Salt and black pepper

Preheat the oven to 350°F | 175°C. Line 3 cups of a standard muffin tin with paper liners, or use 3 small ramekins.

Whisk the eggs in a bowl and set aside.

Heat the oil in a small skillet over medium heat. Add the spinach, tomato, green onion, bell pepper, and garlic and sauté for about 2 minutes, until the spinach wilts. Remove the skillet from the heat and let cool slightly. The vegetables should be cool enough so as not to cook the egg when you stir them together.

Stir the vegetables into the eggs and season with salt and pepper to taste.

Pour the egg mixture evenly into the lined muffin cups or ramekins. Bake for 20 minutes, or until set and golden brown.

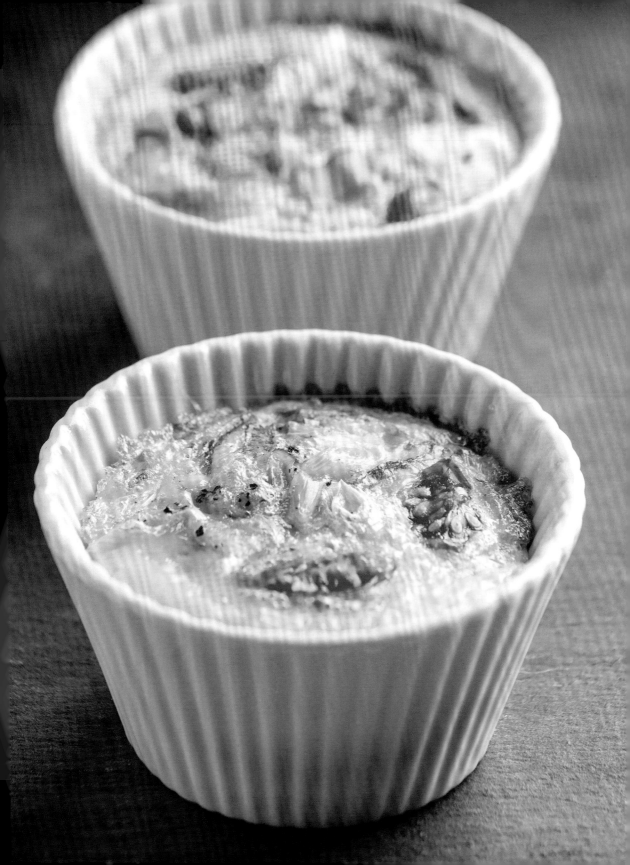

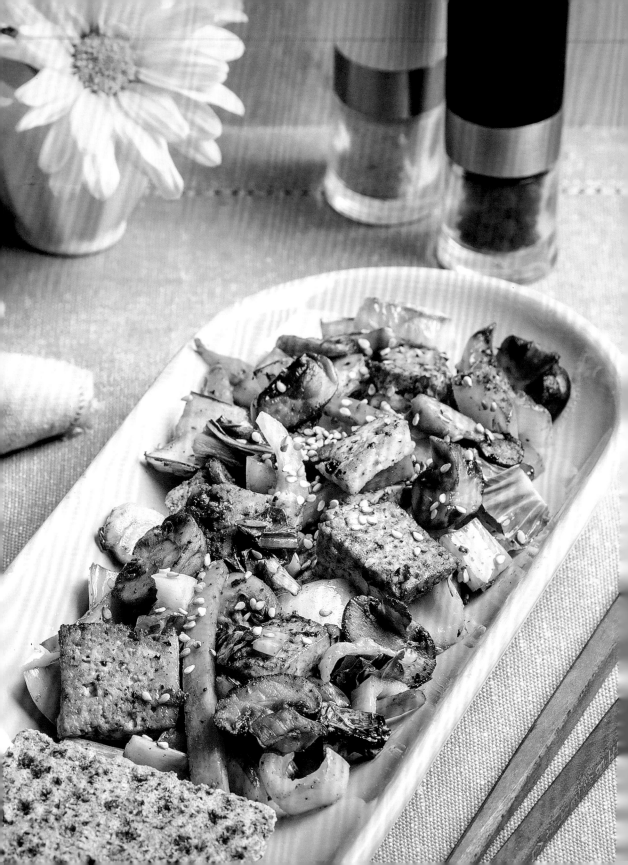

stir-fried veggies
with tofu

Tofu has little flavor on its own, yet it absorbs the flavors of other ingredients, so it's a very versatile protein that goes well with many different accompaniments and seasonings. The black and white sesame seeds sprinkled on top help elevate this dish to something special. Serve with rye crackers, if you like.

Makes 1 serving

1½ oz | 45 g firm tofu

2 tsp | 10 mL coconut or olive oil

½ green onion (white part only), thinly sliced

1 (½-in | 2.5-cm) piece fresh ginger, minced or grated

1 garlic clove, minced

2 button mushrooms, sliced

1 small carrot, julienned

3 leaves baby bok choy, sliced

⅛ tsp chili powder

Salt and black pepper

½ tsp sesame seeds

Press the tofu to remove excess liquid and improve its texture: Put a paper towel on a plate and place the tofu on top. Cover with another paper towel and another plate. Place something heavy on top to weigh it down, like a few books or a can of tomatoes, to press out the extra liquid. Leave the tofu for 15 minutes, changing paper towels if needed. Cut the tofu into 1-in | 2.5-cm cubes.

Heat the oil in a wok over medium-high heat. Add the tofu and cook until seared on all sides, about 5 minutes. Transfer the tofu to a plate.

Add the green onion, ginger, and garlic to the wok and stir-fry until the onion is translucent, about 3 minutes. Stir in the mushrooms, carrot, bok choy, chili powder, and seared tofu and stir-fry until the mushrooms and carrot have softened, about 2 minutes. Season with salt and pepper to taste. Sprinkle with the sesame seeds and serve immediately.

warm strawberry goat cheese spread
with crackers

I eat strawberries every day, preferably organic. I do a lot of hot yoga and their juice is really hydrating. Strawberries also provide powerful antioxidant and anti-inflammatory protection. Think "warm strawberries and cream," and you'll have an idea of how delicious this breakfast is. Substitute veggies for the rye crackers, if you wish.

Makes 1 serving

¾ cup | 110 g
sliced strawberries

¼ cup | 60 mL water

¼ cup | 40 g goat cheese

¼ tsp ground nutmeg

2 rye crackers
(such as Wasa or Ryvita)
or 1 slice rye bread,
toasted

3–4 fresh mint leaves

In a small saucepan, combine the strawberries and water. Cook over medium-low heat until the fruit is soft and slightly thickened and most of the water has evaporated, 5–7 minutes.

Put the goat cheese in a bowl. Stir the warm strawberries and nutmeg into the goat cheese. Spread on the crackers or toast and garnish with the mint.

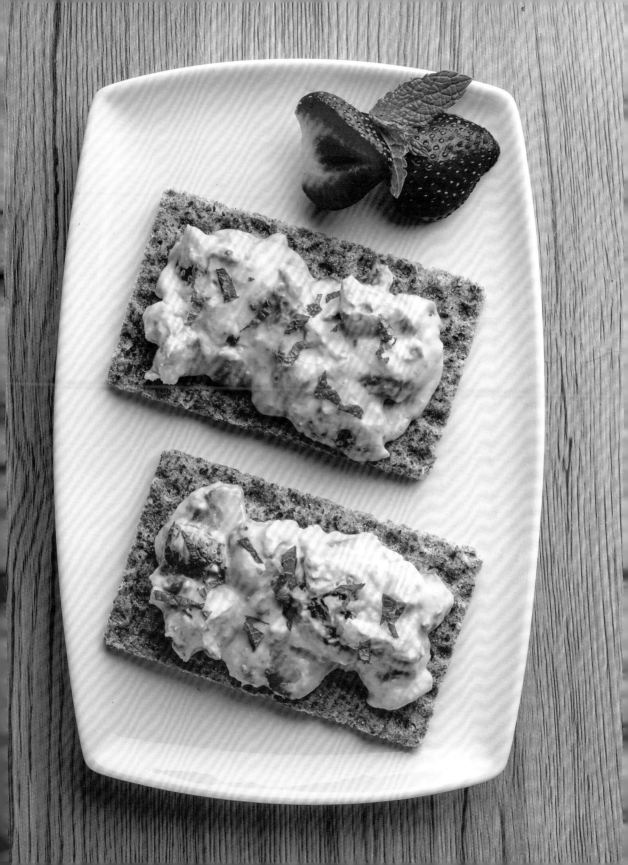

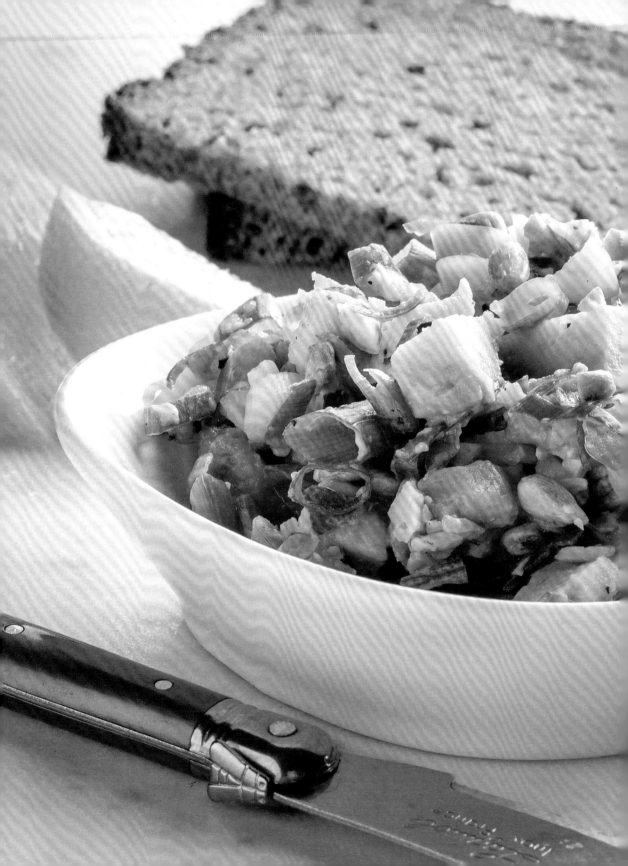

seedy
guacamole spread

australia

Who would think that combining nuts, seeds, garlic, and avocado would taste this good? The garlic gives this breakfast dish, which comes from Metabolic Balance coaches in Australia, such great flavor. Use this spread on rye bread, apple slices, or cut vegetables.

Makes 1 serving

½ avocado

1 green onion, chopped

1 garlic clove, chopped

2 tbsp | 20 g almonds, roughly chopped

2 tbsp | 20 g sunflower seeds

1 tbsp | 15 mL fresh lemon juice

Salt and black pepper

Combine the avocado, green onion, garlic, almonds, sunflower seeds, and lemon juice in a bowl and mash everything together with a fork. Season with salt and pepper to taste. Enjoy immediately.

TIP: If you have leftover spread, you can sprinkle lemon juice on it and cover with plastic wrap to prevent browning of the avocado.

About the Ingredient: Lemon Juice

Lemon juice can cleanse the bloodstream, lower cholesterol, and reduce inflammation, and it serves as a solvent for uric acid buildup, which can cause pain and stiffness in the joints. Lemon juice also helps make your body more alkaline, which can make losing weight easier. In phase 2, lemon would need to be listed as one of your fruits, but you may introduce lemon juice freely during phases 3 or 4. For recipes including lemon juice, remember apple cider vinegar is a great alternative.

Special acknowledgment to Cherry Wills in Australia for this recipe.

Have only 1 complete protein at each meal and eat 3 different protein groups each day.

For your 3 meals each day, it is important to choose a protein so that you are eating from 3 different protein groups. This will help maximize your absorption of nutrients and decrease appetite. The protein groups include meats, fish and other seafood, poultry, dairy (eggs, cheese, milk, yogurt), legumes (including soy products), nuts and seeds, sprouts, and shiitake and oyster mushrooms.

In the digestive tract, our bodies use enzymes to break down the ingested proteins into individual amino acids. Amino acids are the building blocks of protein. They are absorbed through the intestinal wall, where they are reassembled into human proteins. The critical factor for optimum metabolism is not determined by the overall quantity of proteins consumed, but rather by the spectrum of amino acids they contain. The 9 essential amino acids are essential because they cannot be synthesized by the body and therefore need to be ingested as food. The more easily a protein can be converted into highly available protein in the body, the higher its biological value. The usability of a protein is actually decided by the amino acid that is present in the *smallest* quantity. When different protein foods are combined, the biological value is determined by the amino acid whose overall proportion is lowest. Above this level, all other unused amino acids will become waste products in the body, which can lead to increased acidity, as well as other issues.

The ideal amino acid ratio is found in egg yolk, in which 100 percent of the 9 essential amino acids can be converted into human protein. Therefore, egg yolk has a biological value (BV) of 100; BV is a measure of how readily our cells can use the protein from the foods we eat. In contrast, cow's milk has a BV of 91, beef has a BV of 74, and soybeans have a BV of 73, to name a few examples. This is why combining proteins is not recommended: it can actually lower the overall biological value of what you are eating.

Metabolic Balance uses proteins primarily with a high BV (above 70) and recommends eating only one type of protein at each meal. Otherwise, it is possible that the biological value of a protein in a meal will be reduced, resulting in over-acidification of the body.

See pages 34, 39, 65, 131, and 206 for the other Rules of Metabolic Balance!

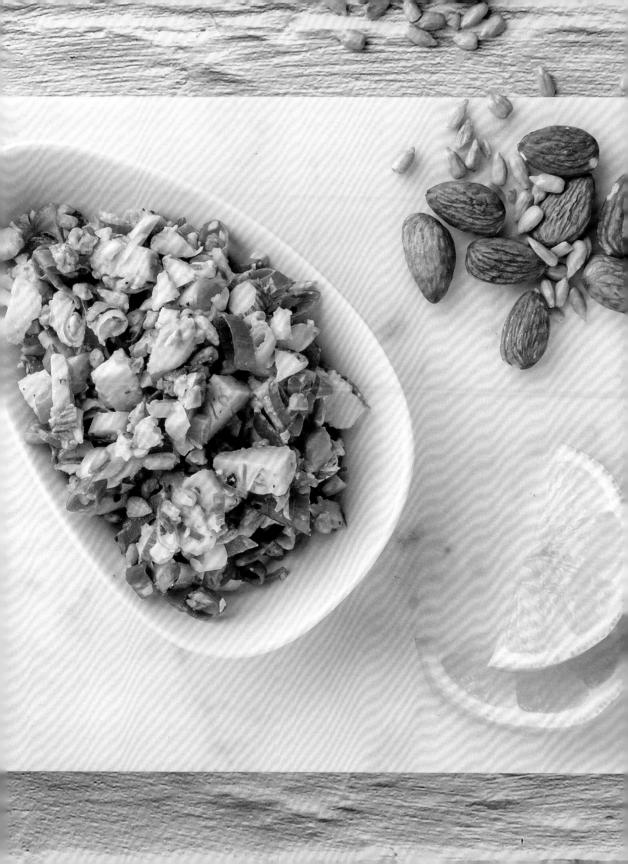

vegetable-herb **spread**

When traveling to international Metabolic Balance conferences, I always look forward to the food—especially the food in Germany, as it is so hearty and nutritionally dense. I know that between meals, I'm not going to be hungry, which always helps me stay on my plan. People always think that when on a weight loss or weight maintenance journey, they won't get enough food—but that is not true with Metabolic Balance. This recipe from the Metabolic Balance coaches in Germany makes a generous portion and has creaminess and crunch from the toasted seeds.

Makes 1 serving

2 tbsp | 20 g
sunflower seeds

2 tbsp | 20 g
pumpkin seeds

¼ tsp vegetable broth
powder

½ avocado,
coarsely chopped

2 cherry tomatoes,
quartered

½ bunch chives,
finely chopped

3 fresh basil leaves,
finely chopped

1 slice rye bread,
toasted, or 2 rye crackers
(such as Wasa or Ryvita)

Salt and black pepper

Put the sunflower and pumpkin seeds in a small bowl and cover with cool water. Stir in the vegetable broth powder and cover the bowl and let the seeds soak overnight on the counter.

In the morning, drain the seeds and set aside 1 tbsp | 16 g for toasting.

In a medium bowl, mix the remaining seeds, the avocado, tomatoes, chives, and basil and stir.

In a small nonstick skillet, toast the reserved seeds over medium-high heat until any residual moisture has evaporated and some start jumping in the pan, like popcorn.

Spread the avocado mixture on the bread or crackers, season with salt and pepper to taste, and top with the toasted seeds.

Special acknowledgment to Silvia Bürkle in Germany for this recipe.

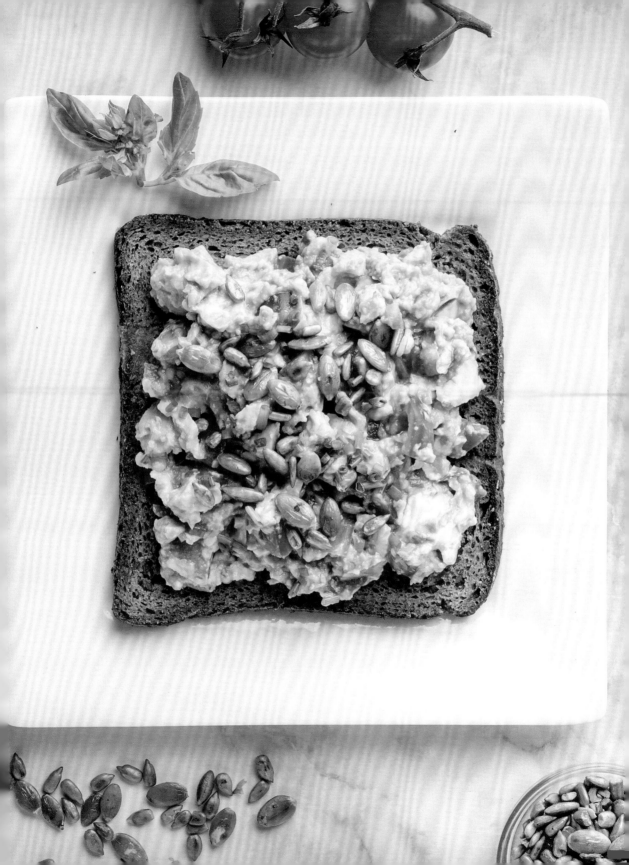

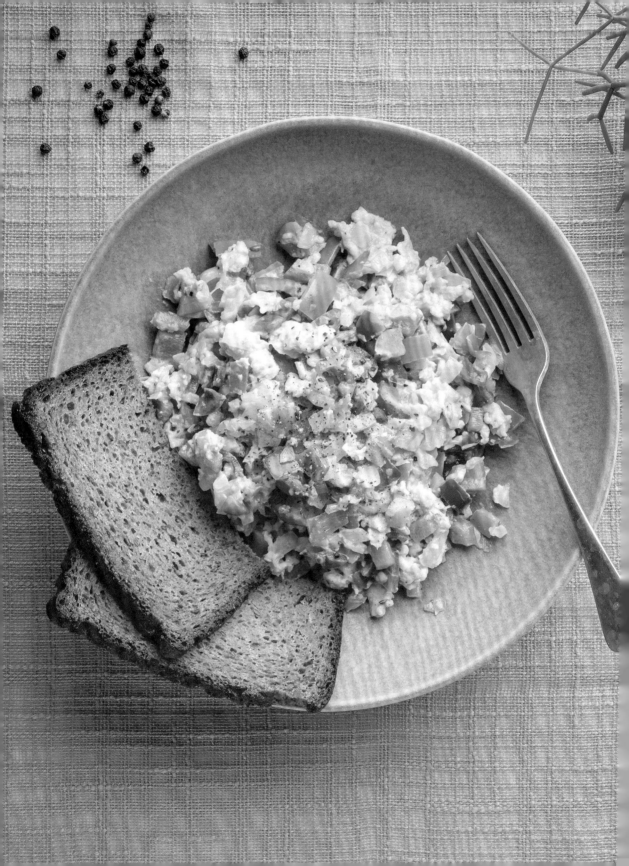

menemen (scrambled eggs with tomato)

Menemen, made from eggs, tomatoes, and sometimes peppers, is a very common breakfast dish in Turkey. It will start your engine on a chilly winter morning when you want to stay in bed, and it's hearty enough to keep you satisfied until lunchtime. I'm glad the Metabolic Balance coaches in Turkey shared this dish, as it is a new favorite of mine. Serve it with rye bread while still warm.

Makes 1 serving

2 large eggs

2 tbsp | 30 mL olive oil

1 small onion, chopped

1 long green bell pepper, chopped

½ tsp salt

1 small tomato, chopped

Pinch black pepper (optional)

1 tbsp chopped fresh parsley

Whisk the eggs in a bowl and set aside.

Heat the oil in a medium skillet over medium-low heat. Add the onion and sauté until it begins to soften, 2–3 minutes. Stir in the green pepper and salt, cover, and cook, stirring occasionally, until the pepper is soft, about 2 minutes. Stir in the tomato, cover, and cook until the tomato is soft, 3 minutes.

Pour in the eggs and stir to incorporate. Cook, stirring occasionally, until the eggs are lightly scrambled, about 3 minutes.

Sprinkle black pepper on top, if you like, and garnish with the parsley.

The 8 Rules of Metabolic Balance: Rule #4
Always begin each meal with two bites of protein.

Always begin each meal with one or two bites of protein to have a longer-lasting effect on your insulin levels. When the stomach receives protein first, the pancreas reacts by secreting the hormone glucagon. This hormone is the antagonist of insulin, which means that it blocks insulin production and also triggers a feeling of satiety. The result is a lower insulin level, which stimulates fat burning, blocks fat synthesis, and prevents hunger.

See pages 34, 39, 60, 131, and 206 for the other Rules of Metabolic Balance!

BREAKFASTS

Special acknowledgment to Sophie Kamuran Demirtas in Turkey for this recipe.

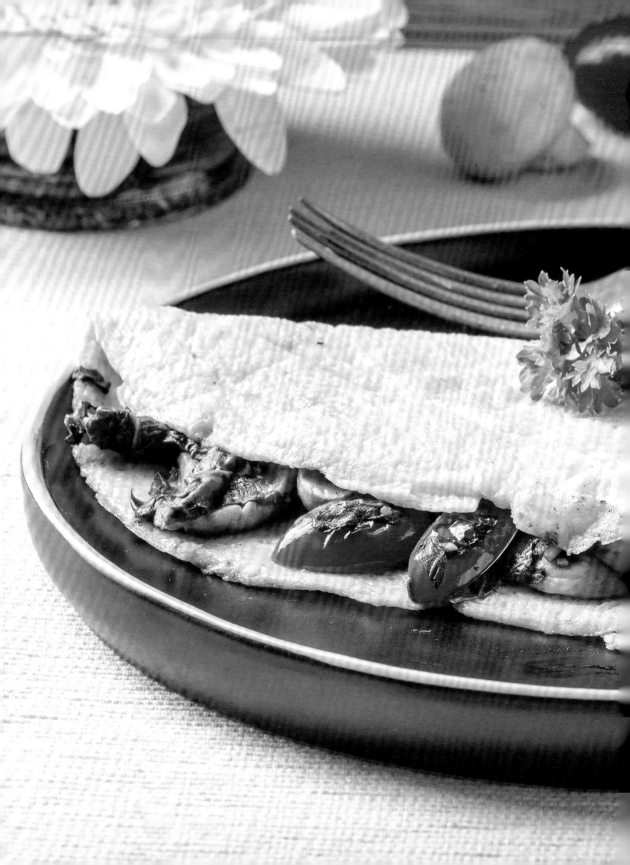

ultimate veggie omelet

Finding ways to make delicious dishes can be challenging in the morning, when many of us are pressed for time before work. This omelet is quick and delicious and elevates your morning routine to new heights. The smell of frying garlic awakens my senses and reminds me of great home cooking. For a full meal, enjoy this with rye crackers and a serving of fruit.

Makes 1 serving

2 large eggs

1 tbsp | 15 mL olive oil, divided

1 large handful baby spinach, roughly chopped

1 small tomato, quartered

2 button mushrooms, sliced

1 small garlic clove, minced or grated

½ tsp salt

Chopped fresh parsley, for garnish (optional)

Whisk the eggs in a bowl and set aside.

Put 1 tsp | 5mL of the oil in a medium nonstick skillet and spread to coat. Heat over medium heat. Add the spinach, tomato, mushrooms, garlic, and salt and sauté 2–3 minutes, or until the spinach is wilted and the mushrooms are soft. Transfer the vegetables to a bowl.

Add the remaining 2 tsp | 10 mL oil to the skillet. Pour in the eggs and cook on medium heat until set on the bottom, 3–5 minutes. Then flip and continue to cook until completely set, 1–2 minutes more. Spread the veggie mixture over half of the omelet, then fold over the other half to cover. Garnish with parsley, if desired, and serve immediately.

spinach and mushroom frittata

Mushrooms have a natural umami flavor that enhances the taste of any food with which they are cooked. *Umami* means "essence of deliciousness" in Japanese, and its taste is described as a meaty, savory quality that deepens flavor. This single-serving frittata has a wonderful flavor from mushrooms and dried herbs. I like to use Italian seasoning blend, but you could instead use dried oregano, basil, parsley, or thyme, depending on what's in your spice cabinet.

Makes 1 serving

2 large eggs

⅛ tsp dried Italian seasoning blend

Salt and black pepper to taste

2 tbsp | 30 mL vegetable broth

1 small handful baby spinach, chopped

2 button mushrooms, chopped

Preheat the oven to 375°F | 190°C.

In a small bowl, whisk the eggs, herbs, and salt and pepper to taste. Set aside.

In a small saucepan, heat the vegetable broth over medium heat. Add the spinach and mushrooms and cook until the spinach has wilted, about 2 minutes. Transfer to a bowl to cool slightly.

Add the spinach and mushrooms to the egg mixture and stir until well mixed.

Pour the mixture into a small baking dish. Bake for 10 minutes, or until browned and set.

Let cool for 5 minutes, then serve.

Pictured on page 32

mild curry omelet

I love the flavor of curry, and this delicately spiced omelet lets me enjoy it at breakfast too. Turmeric is warm and bittersweet. It has powerful anti-inflammatory properties, has been found to promote optimal liver function, and is rich in iron and manganese.

Makes 1 serving

2 large eggs

1 tbsp | 15 mL coconut or olive oil

1 small garlic clove, minced

1 small onion, diced

½ red bell pepper, diced

¼ tsp salt

1 small handful baby spinach

2–3 cilantro sprigs, chopped

½ tsp ground cumin

½ tsp ground turmeric

Whisk the eggs in a bowl and set aside.

Heat the oil in a small skillet over medium heat. Add the garlic and sauté until fragrant, about 20 seconds. Stir in the onion, bell pepper, and salt. Sauté until the vegetables soften, 1–2 minutes. Toss in the spinach and cilantro and continue to cook until wilted. Sprinkle with the cumin and turmeric and cook until fragrant, about 30 seconds. Spread the vegetables evenly over the bottom of the pan.

Pour in the eggs and cook until set, then flip the omelet and cook for an additional 30 seconds to set the other side.

Roll the omelet onto a plate or fold in half to serve.

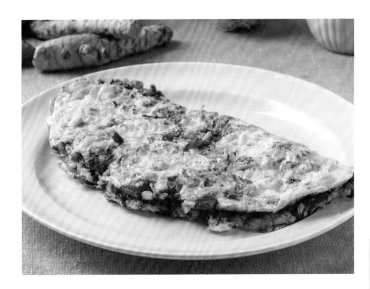

oat pudding with
spicy mango chutney

france

Do you think that oatmeal is only a cold-weather food? Wait until you try this chilled oat pudding! This breakfast, which comes from Metabolic Balance coaches in France, is bursting with flavor and fills you right up. The fresh flavors of the mango chutney add a sweet and savory punch. This dish is also loaded with fiber—a bonus for your digestive health. This recipe makes enough for 2 servings, so it's great to share, or you can keep the second portion in the fridge to enjoy another day.

Makes 2 servings

Pudding

1¾ cups | 415 mL whole milk

⅓ vanilla bean

1 cinnamon stick

1 cup | 100 g rolled oats

2 tbsp | 23 g whole chia seeds

Unsweetened shaved coconut, for garnish (optional)

Chutney

2 medium ripe mangoes

1 (1-in | 2.5-cm) piece fresh ginger, grated (to taste)

¼ tsp ground sumac or grated lemon zest

¼ tsp ground turmeric

¼ tsp ground cumin

In a small saucepan, bring the milk to a boil, then lower the heat to a simmer. Split the vanilla bean and scrape the seeds into the pan, then add the pod itself. Add the cinnamon stick. Simmer for 10 minutes. Remove the pan from the heat and set aside to cool.

Once the milk has cooled, remove the skin from the surface and pour the milk (along with the vanilla pod and cinnamon stick) into a medium bowl. Add the oats and chia seeds and mix well with a wooden spoon. Cover and refrigerate overnight.

Peel and pit the mangoes, then chop the flesh into small cubes. Transfer to a small bowl. Add the ginger, sumac, turmeric, and cumin. Cover the bowl and refrigerate overnight.

In the morning, remove the cinnamon stick and vanilla pod from the pudding. Divide the pudding between two bowls or large glasses. Top with the mango chutney. Add the shaved coconut on top, if desired.

Special acknowledgment to Laurent Causse in France for this recipe.

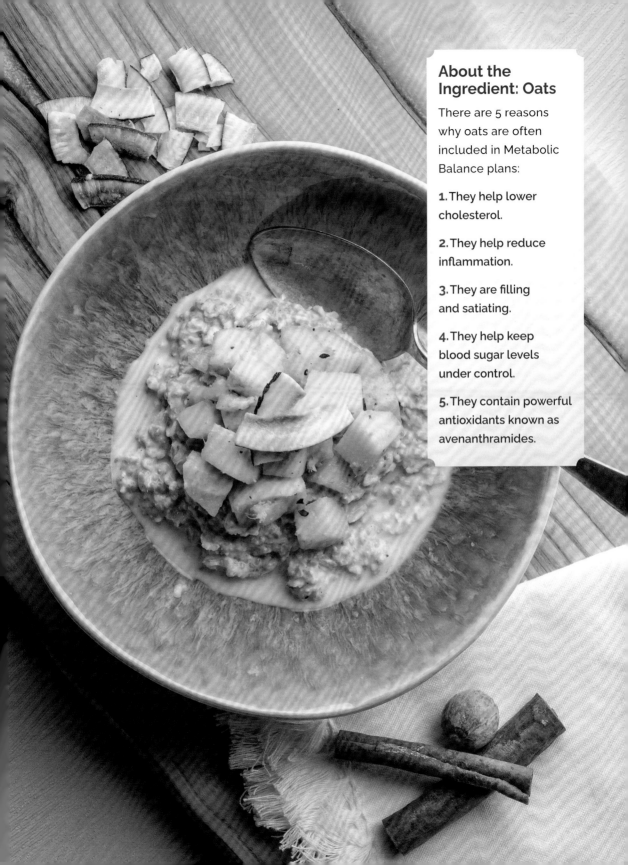

About the Ingredient: Oats

There are 5 reasons why oats are often included in Metabolic Balance plans:

1. They help lower cholesterol.

2. They help reduce inflammation.

3. They are filling and satiating.

4. They help keep blood sugar levels under control.

5. They contain powerful antioxidants known as avenanthramides.

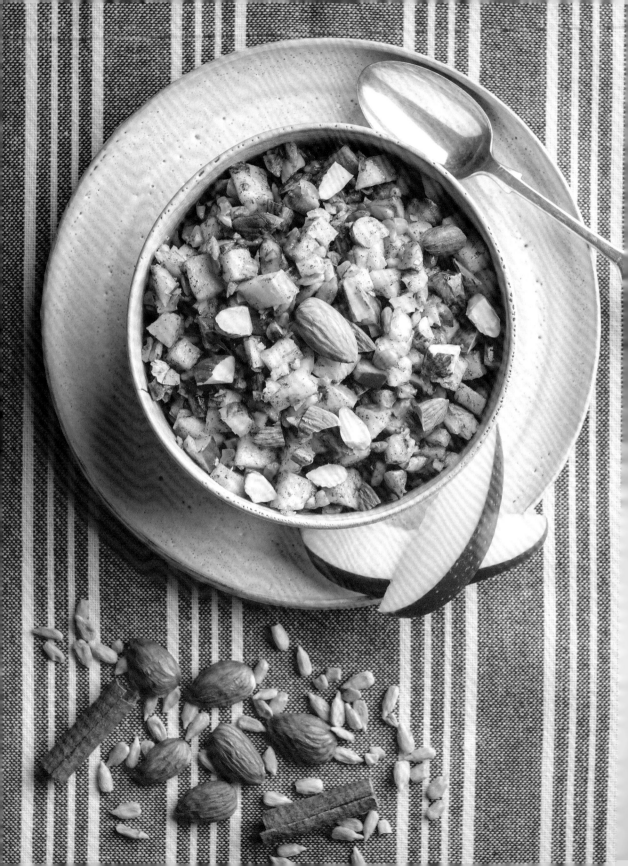

mandelade
with chopped fruit

Mandel is German for "almond," and mandelade is a classic Metabolic Balance breakfast consisting of soaked nuts and seeds combined with chopped fruit (in this case, apple, but you can substitute pear or berries, or whatever fruit is on your personal plan, if you have one). I like it with Red Delicious, Granny Smith, or Royal Gala apples, but choose any tart apple you like to eat. Soaking the almonds and sunflower seeds makes them easier to digest, which increases the absorption of nutrients. Try this for breakfast using whole, raw almonds with the skins for added dietary fiber, vitamins, and minerals. Mandelade can be served cool after prepping the ingredients or baked in muffin cups and served warm (see the variation below).

Makes 1 serving

3 tbsp | 30 g almonds

2 tbsp | 20 g sunflower seeds

1 medium apple, cored and finely chopped

¼ tsp ground cinnamon

Put the almonds and sunflower seeds in a small bowl and cover with cool water. Cover the bowl and let the nuts and seeds soak overnight on the counter.

In the morning, drain the nuts and seeds and finely chop them. Transfer to a small bowl and stir in the apple and cinnamon.

Warm Version: Preheat the oven to 400°F | 205°C. Line 4 cups of a standard muffin tin with paper liners. Spoon the mixture into the lined muffin cups and bake for 15 minutes, or until the edges are golden brown. Enjoy warm.

TIP: You can pulse the almonds and sunflower seeds with the apple in a food processor, but take care not to over-chop.

cinnamon
apple pancakes

As children, for an occasional Sunday family treat, we would go to our local Golden Griddle pancake house. Marshaling 9 hungry and excited children was a sight to behold. The smell of pancakes was comforting to us, and our parents could hardly believe how much we could eat. Thanks to the Canadian Metabolic Balance coaches for these delicious and filling rye pancakes. The softened apple and cinnamon provide enough sweetness to satisfy any cravings you might have—especially when served with fresh berries or other low glycemic load fruits.

Makes 1 serving

1 large egg

2 tbsp | 16 g rye flour

1 tsp baking powder

½ tsp | 2.5 mL vanilla extract

½ tsp ground cinnamon

Pinch salt

2 tbsp | 30 mL water

1 medium apple, cored and sliced into 4–5 rounds

1 tsp | 5 mL coconut oil

In a bowl, whisk the egg and then add the rye flour, baking powder, vanilla, cinnamon, and salt. Combine thoroughly. Set aside.

Heat the water in a medium skillet over medium heat. Add the apple slices, cover, and steam until softened, 3–4 minutes. Carefully transfer the apples to a plate and wipe out any remaining water from the pan.

Return the pan to the heat and add the oil. Return the apple slices to the pan, making sure they are not overlapping. Spoon an equal amount of rye batter over each slice. After about 2 minutes, the batter will have set. Carefully flip the pancakes and continue cooking until lightly browned, another 2–3 minutes. Transfer to a plate and serve.

Special acknowledgment to Vera Jamin-Wirth in Canada for this recipe.

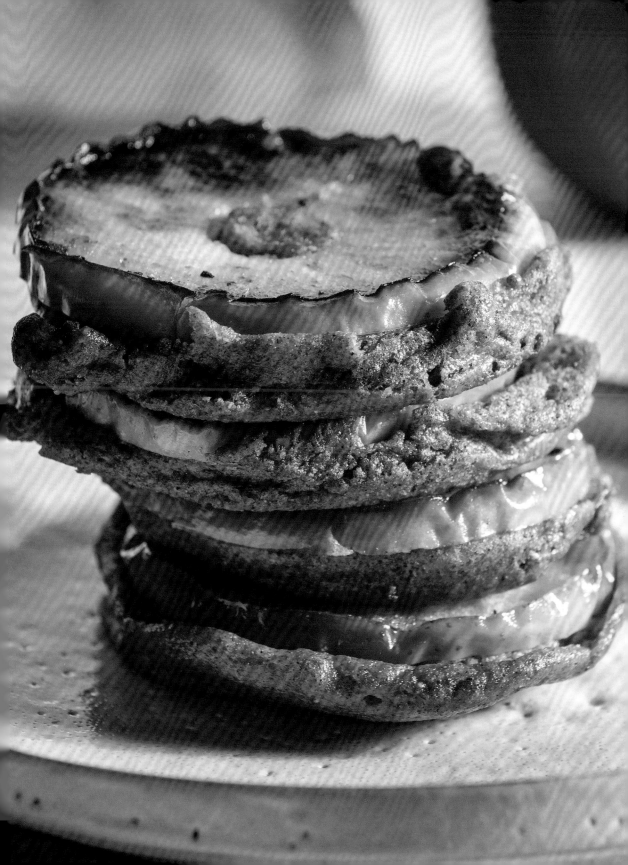

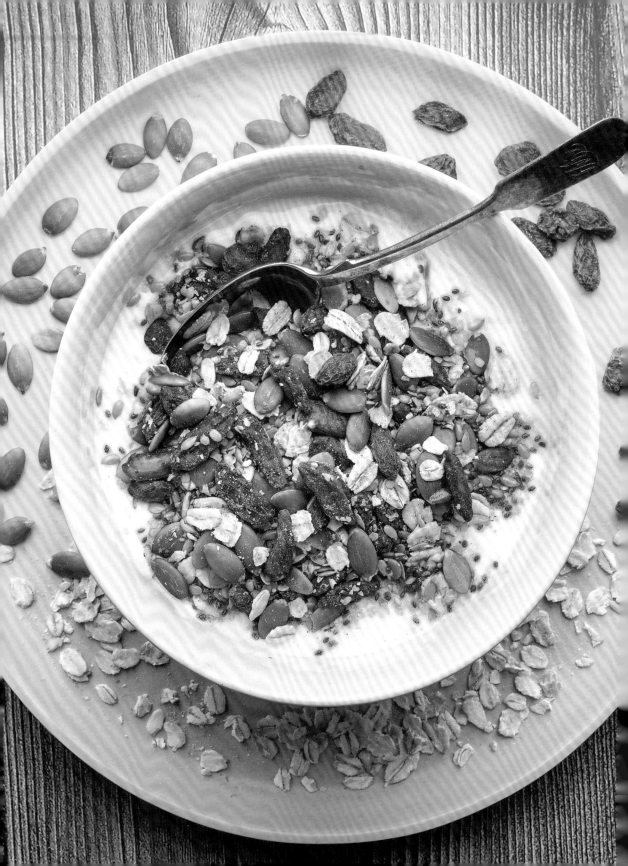

cherry island retreat granola

treat meal

While sitting around a campfire in Northern Ontario at a leadership retreat and deciding what we'd have for breakfast, one participant described this delicious, easy granola recipe. She had brought enough to share with us all, and it became our staple breakfast for the next few days, keeping us full and content. Add 2–3 heaping tablespoons of this granola to your morning yogurt and enjoy!

Makes 8–12 servings

½ cup | 68 g
chia seeds

½ cup | 68 g
flaxseeds

½ cup | 68 g
pumpkin seeds

½ cup | 68 g
steel-cut oats

½ cup | 68 g
hemp hearts

½ cup | 50 g
goji berries

¼ cup | 22 g
oat bran

1 heaping tbsp
ground cinnamon

Mix all the ingredients in a large bowl. Store in a sealed container in the refrigerator.

About the Ingredient: Flaxseeds

Flaxseeds are tiny nutritional powerhouses! They are loaded with heart-healthy omega-3 fatty acids, absorb 8 times their weight, pull toxic metabolites out of the large intestine, make you feel full, contain soluble fiber to regulate blood sugar, prevent constipation, and are a good source of thiamine, copper, magnesium, and phosphorus. Flaxseeds should be ground to allow you to better obtain all their nutritional benefits. However, I do recommend you purchase the seeds whole. Whole seeds will stay fresher for longer at room temperature, and you can easily grind them at home using a coffee grinder or spice mill. Once ground, always keep them in the freezer so they stay fresh.

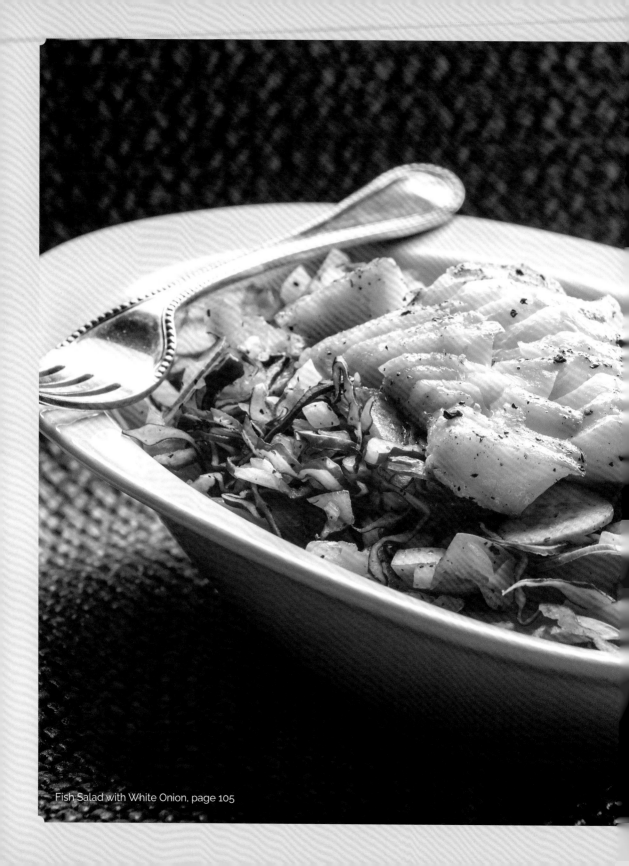

Fish Salad with White Onion, page 105

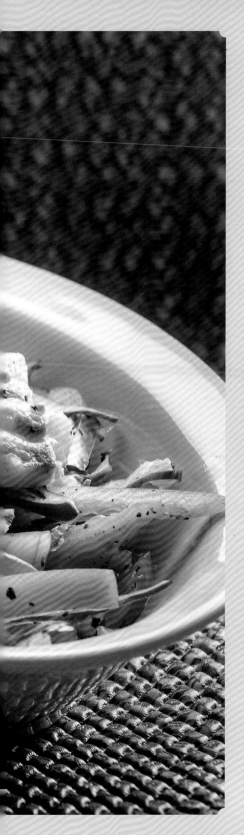

salads

For midday meals, I like to focus on colorful foods that will help me maintain energy until dinnertime. Salads are easy to prepare, and their bright colors and varied textures make them a treat to eat all year long. Though the word *salad* often conjures thoughts of bowls of raw greens, you can make salads from a wide variety of leaves, stalks, stems, and flowers, enjoyed cold or warm, which makes them a great foundation to build a complete and nutritious meal. I crave salads and sometimes have salads for both lunch and dinner. I just love the freshness and varied tastes of salads, not to mention their many health benefits. Choosing the right plant foods as your base means your salad can be loaded with antioxidants, which protect your body from disease, and fiber, which keeps you feeling full and satisfied.

arugula and salmon **salad**

I could eat arugula and salmon every day! The pungent and slightly bitter arugula complements the sweet and salty salmon, and the dill gives it extra zest. This richly flavored and brightly colored salad is so inviting!

Makes 1 serving

4½ oz | 130 g salmon

1 tbsp | 15 mL soy sauce

Juice of 1 lemon

1 tsp | 5 mL ghee

1 cup | 20 g arugula

2 tbsp | 10 g finely chopped red onion

2 tbsp | 10 g finely chopped celery

2 tbsp | 10 g thinly sliced red bell pepper

1 tbsp finely chopped fresh dill

2 tsp | 10 mL olive oil

1 tsp | 5 mL balsamic vinegar

Salt and black pepper

Set the salmon in a shallow bowl. In a small bowl, mix together the soy sauce and lemon juice. Pour over the salmon and set aside to marinate for 15–20 minutes (no more or the acid in the lemon juice will "cook" the fish).

Heat the ghee in a small skillet over medium heat. Add the salmon and sear until cooked through, about 2 minutes on each side. Transfer to a plate and let cool. When cool enough to handle, break the salmon into bite-size pieces.

In a bowl, toss together the arugula, red onion, celery, and bell pepper. Top with the salmon, sprinkle with the dill, and drizzle with the oil and vinegar. Season with salt and pepper to taste.

About the Ingredient: Arugula

Arugula is a salad green that is also known as rocket or rucola. Its taste is a bit peppery and nutty. It has a high sulfur content and is an excellent internal cleanser and liver purifier.

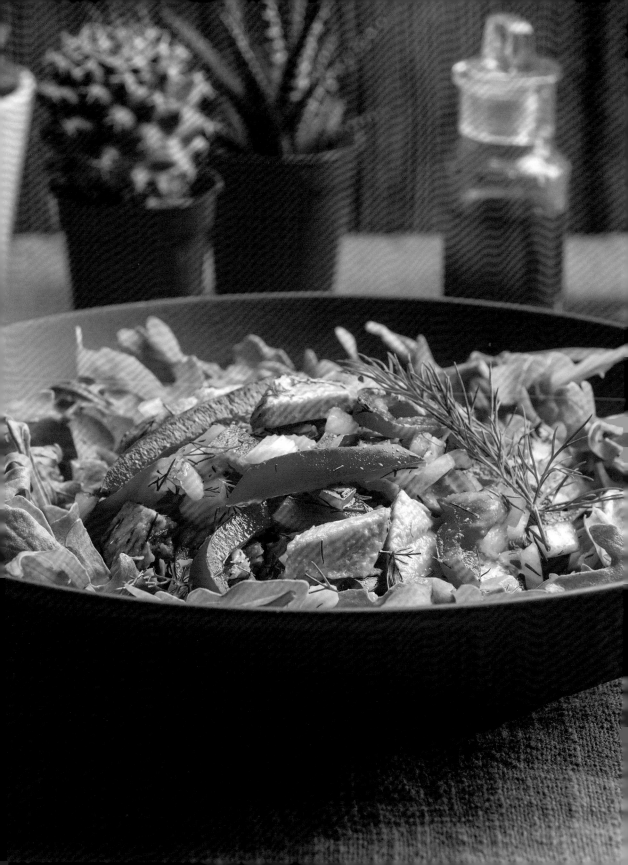

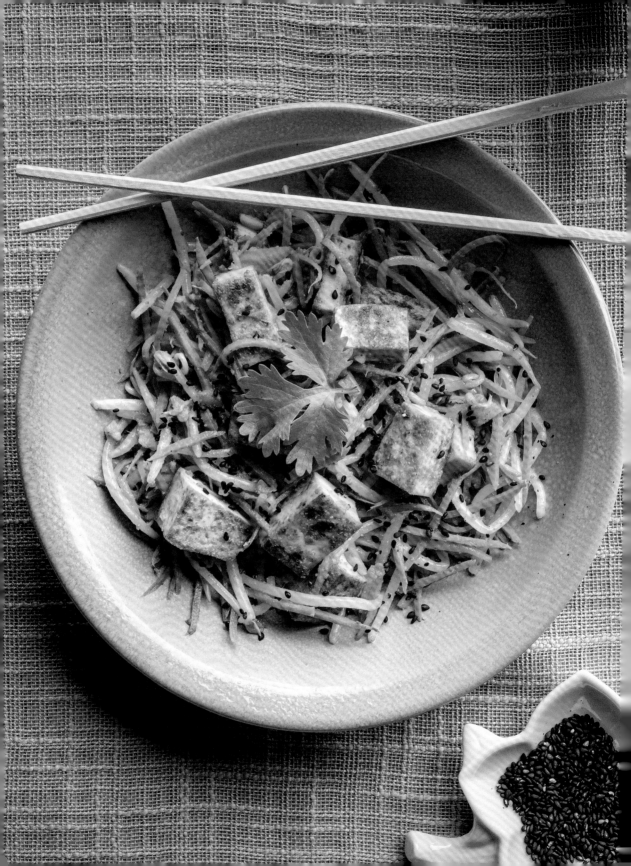

warm curried carrot salad
with tofu

Because of carrots' abundance of essential vitamins, minerals, and antioxidants, many nutrition experts award this humble veggie superfood status. Carrots are a carotenoid-rich food, and eating them with nuts or oil maximizes the absorption of beta-carotene. Antioxidants like beta-carotene help reduce or prevent oxidative stress in the body, which is known to contribute to the development of chronic diseases. Beta-carotene can even improve cognitive function, according to some studies.

Makes 1 serving

3 oz | 85 g firm tofu

2 tsp | 10 mL coconut oil

1 cup | 65 g zucchini, sliced into long, thin strips

1 small carrot, grated

1 (1-in | 2.5-cm) piece fresh ginger, grated

½ tsp curry powder

Salt and black pepper

½ tsp black and white sesame seeds, for garnish

Chopped fresh cilantro, for garnish

Press the tofu to remove excess liquid and improve its texture: Put a paper towel on a plate and place the tofu on top. Cover with another paper towel and another plate. Place something heavy on top to weigh it down, like a few books or a can of tomatoes, to press out the extra liquid. Leave the tofu for 15 minutes, changing paper towels if needed. Cut the tofu into ½-in | 2.5-cm slices.

Heat the oil in a small skillet over medium heat. Add the tofu, zucchini, carrot, and ginger and stir-fry until the carrot softens, about 2 minutes. Season with the curry powder and salt and pepper to taste. Stir-fry until the tofu is firm and starts to brown and the carrot and zucchini are soft, 3–5 minutes.

Transfer to a plate to cool slightly, then garnish with the sesame seeds and cilantro.

Note: To make this a high-protein treat meal, swap the zucchini for an equal amount of bean sprouts (as pictured).

avocado chicken salad

This creamy, delicious chicken salad is super easy to prepare, especially if you already have cooked chicken on hand—making this an excellent recipe to use up leftovers from last night's chicken dinner. Spread the chicken salad on rye bread or rye crackers or pile it in a lettuce wrap for a delicious meal.

Makes 1 serving

3½ oz | 100 g cooked boneless, skinless chicken breast

½ avocado, diced

1 tbsp | 15 mL fresh lime juice

½ tsp chili powder

Salt and black pepper

½ celery rib, chopped

1 green onion, chopped

Chopped fresh cilantro, for garnish

Cut the chicken breast into bite-size pieces.

In a medium bowl, use a fork to mash half of the avocado with the lime juice, chili powder, and salt and pepper to taste until creamy. Add the chicken to the bowl of mashed avocado and mix well. Add the remaining avocado, celery, and green onion, and give everything a light toss. Garnish with cilantro.

About the Ingredient: Avocado

Although they are usually served in savory preparations like vegetables, and they are considered vegetables on the Metabolic Balance program, avocados are actually tropical fruits. Avocados are rich in oleic acid, with 59 percent of their fat content in heart-healthy monosaturated fat. They are loaded with potassium, a mineral that helps regulate blood pressure.

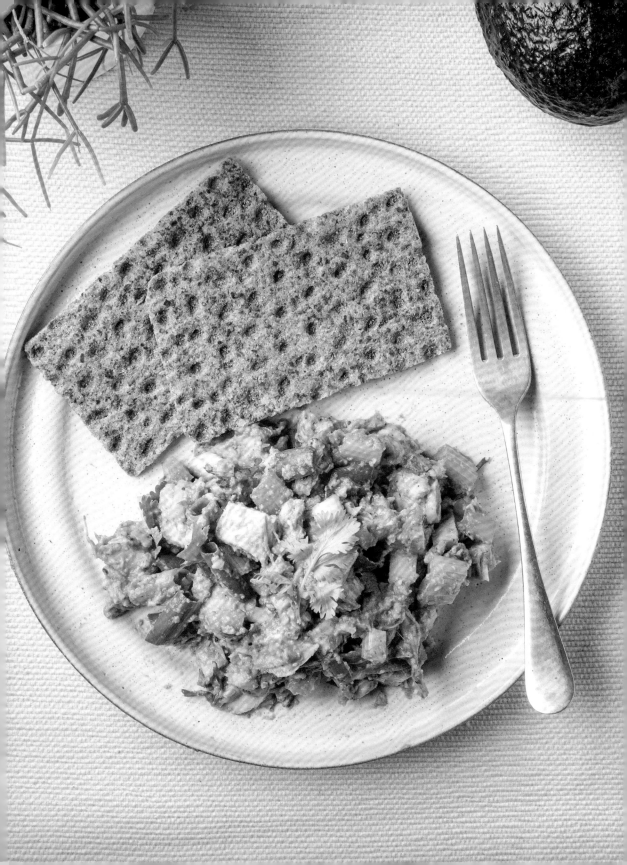

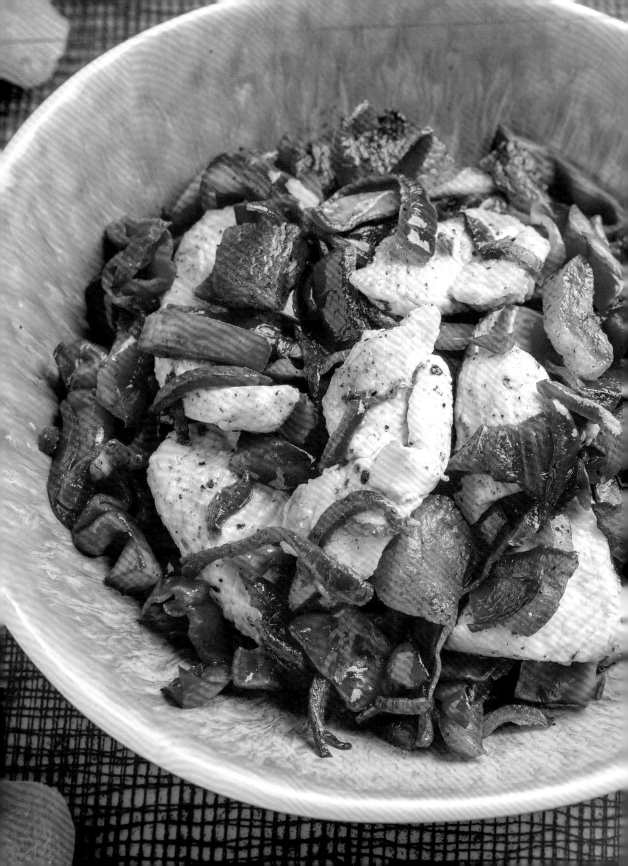

sweet and savory
red cabbage salad with apricots and turkey

In the US and Canada, many people think that cabbage is good for only one thing: coleslaw. But this neglected vegetable offers so much more and can be enjoyed raw or cooked, in salads, slaws, soups, dumplings, stir-fries—the list goes on. While both green and red cabbage are full of nutrients that aid in digestion, red cabbage has a vibrant hue that adds a lovely pop of color to many dishes. When I made this dish the first time, I was saving it for my next day's lunch, only to discover that my husband had taken it. He asked for more the next day! The apricots give this warm salad some sweetness and added texture, and the nutmeg and allspice add a "Grandma's home cooking" flavor.

Makes 1 serving

4½ oz | 130 g boneless, skinless turkey breast

Salt and black pepper

1 tbsp | 15 mL olive oil, divided

⅓ red onion, thinly sliced

⅛ tsp ground allspice

⅛ tsp ground nutmeg

4 red cabbage leaves, thinly sliced

4 dried apricots, sliced

4 tsp | 20 mL balsamic vinegar

Cut the turkey into bite-size pieces and transfer to a small bowl. Season with salt and pepper to taste and toss to coat.

In a medium skillet, heat half of the oil over medium-high heat. Add the turkey and sauté until cooked through, about 10 minutes. Transfer the turkey to a bowl.

Add the remaining olive oil to the skillet. Add the onion, allspice, and nutmeg and stir-fry for 1 minute. Add the cabbage and apricots and sauté until well coated, about 2 minutes. Add the vinegar and toss until juices are reduced to a glaze and the cabbage is crisp-tender, about 6 minutes.

Transfer the vegetable mixture to the bowl with the turkey and toss to combine.

garlic **caesar salad**

While white-bread croutons make this salad a definite treat meal, it is one of my signature dishes and I had to include it in this book. I have been making this recipe since my children were young and still volunteer to make it for every family occasion. If I don't come with this salad, I hear about it! When I bring it to Sunday dinners with my grandkids, my granddaughters always lick the bowl. My sister-in-law, Jennifer, begs me to bring her a bottle of this dressing for Christmas Eve every year. Having a family of 100 people, when I make it for the whole crew, that's a lot of lettuce! This recipe makes just enough to serve 2 or 3 people.

Makes 2–3 servings

Chicken

2 (5-oz | 140-g) boneless, skinless chicken breasts

Juice of 1 lemon

2 tbsp | 30 mL olive oil

1 tbsp | 15 mL Dijon mustard

Croutons

½ baguette, cut into 1-in | 2.5-cm cubes

3 tbsp | 45 mL olive oil

½ tsp garlic powder

Salt and black pepper

Arrange the chicken breasts in a shallow baking dish. In a small bowl, whisk together the lemon juice, oil, and mustard. Pour over the chicken breasts and turn to coat. Cover the dish and let the chicken marinate in the refrigerator for at least 1 hour, or overnight.

Toward the end of the marinating time, preheat the oven to 350°F | 175°C. Bake the chicken for 30 minutes or until cooked through.

In a large bowl, toss the bread cubes with the oil, garlic powder, and salt and pepper to taste. Spread out the bread cubes on a rimmed baking sheet and bake for 20 minutes (you can put them in the oven with the chicken), turning halfway through. (The croutons can also be made ahead of time and stored in an airtight container.)

Remove everything from the oven. When the chicken is cool enough to handle, slice it against the grain.

Ingredients and directions continued on next page ▸

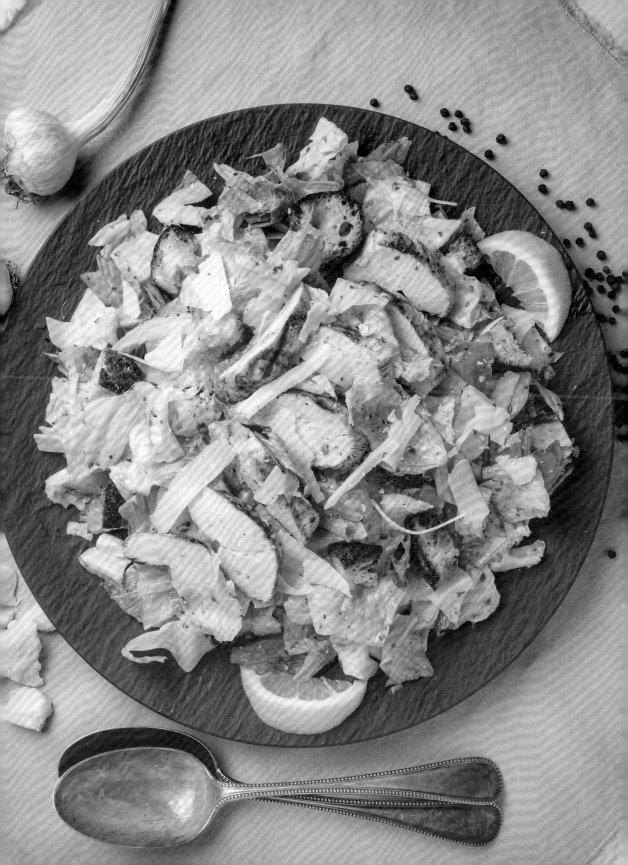

Dressing and Salad

1 large egg

1 bunch curly parsley

Juice of 1 lemon

½ cup | 45 g grated
Parmesan cheese

1 (2-oz | 55-g) can
anchovy fillets in oil

¾ cup | 180 mL olive oil

2 tbsp | 30 mL
Worcestershire sauce

2 tbsp | 30 mL
red wine vinegar

2 tbsp | 30 mL
Dijon mustard

3–6 garlic cloves, peeled

Salt and black pepper

1 head romaine lettuce,
chopped

Meanwhile, make the dressing. To coddle (parboil) the egg, bring a small saucepan of water to a boil. Fill a bowl with cold water and ice.

Add the egg to the boiling water and boil for 1 minute. Immediately transfer the egg to the ice bath for 1–2 minutes. (Coddling reduces the risk of bacterial contamination from a raw egg.)

Crack the egg into a blender or food processor. Add the parsley, lemon juice, Parmesan, anchovies with oil, olive oil, Worcestershire sauce, vinegar, mustard, and garlic and puree until smooth. Season with salt and pepper to taste.

Put the lettuce in a large bowl. Add half of the dressing and toss well. (Store the remaining dressing in an airtight container in the refrigerator for up to 1 week.) Add the chicken and croutons.

The Role of Stress in Health and How to Destress

We all have a little stress in life, but in today's world, people are experiencing prolonged and intense stress, which can cause weight gain, anxiety, depression, sleep problems, digestive issues, and headaches, just to name a few side effects. When you are under constant stress, the hormone cortisol is released. Cortisol increases sugar in the bloodstream, depletes the immune system's resistance, and increases vulnerability to all kinds of illnesses. Finding a solution to stress can be challenging, but managing it is critical for optimal health. Staying positive and finding something you love to do is extremely beneficial to reducing stress. Walking, reading, exercising, eating a healthy diet, getting enough sleep, and re-examining relationships can also help tremendously. My personal philosophy is:

S: Sleep

T: Talk to someone

R: Relax

E: Exercise

S: Self-love

S: Slow down

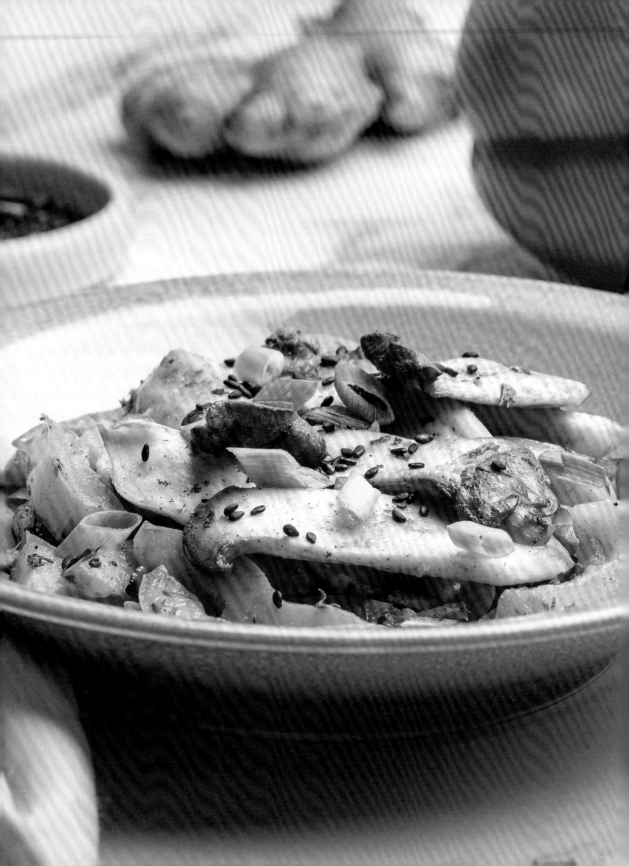

oyster mushrooms
with ginger glaze

Oyster mushrooms can be white, cream, yellow, or reddish brown in color. They have a tender, velvety texture and a savory anise flavor. This dish gets a kick from the ginger and from a dash of hot sauce in the glaze. I like to use Tabasco, but you could also try sriracha or whatever hot sauce you fancy.

Makes 1 serving

4½ oz | 130 g
oyster mushrooms

½ orange bell pepper, sliced

1 (1-in | 2.5-cm) piece fresh ginger, minced

Dash hot sauce

Salt and black pepper

¼ tsp ground turmeric

⅔ cup | 160 mL vegetable broth

1 green onion, sliced on the diagonal, for garnish

½ tsp black sesame seeds, for garnish

Clean any dirt off the mushrooms with a paper towel or the edge of a knife, but don't wash them with water. Cut the mushrooms into thin slices.

Heat a nonstick skillet over medium heat. Add the bell pepper and stir-fry until softened, 1–2 minutes. Transfer the bell pepper to a plate.

Add the mushrooms and ginger to the pan and stir-fry until the mushrooms are softened, about 5 minutes. Add the hot sauce and season with salt and pepper to taste. Add the turmeric and pour in the vegetable broth. Bring to a boil for 2–3 minutes, and add the bell pepper. Stir and then remove from the heat. Garnish with the green onion and sesame seeds.

light and fresh
mushroom sauté

Oyster mushrooms provide several health benefits, including enhancing heart health, protecting the immune system, and encouraging balanced blood sugar. They also provide anti-inflammatory and antioxidant benefits. This dish packs a lot of flavors with the variety of spices. Serve this sauté over a bed of fresh, crisp greens.

Makes 1 serving

4½ oz | 130 g oyster (or shiitake) mushrooms

2 tbsp | 30 mL vegetable broth

½ medium onion, cut into small dice

2 tsp dried tarragon

½ tsp ground nutmeg

¼ tsp salt

¼ tsp black pepper

2 tbsp finely chopped fresh parsley

Clean any dirt off the mushrooms with a paper towel or the edge of a knife, but don't wash them with water. Cut the mushrooms into thin slices.

Heat the vegetable broth in a medium nonstick skillet over medium heat. Add the mushrooms, onion, tarragon, nutmeg, salt, and pepper. Sauté until the mushrooms are tender, about 10 minutes. Stir in the parsley and serve over greens.

About the Ingredient: Mushrooms

On many personalized Metabolic Balance plans, oyster and shiitake mushrooms are listed as a protein. That is because they contain all 9 essential amino acids. They are fabulous for a more plant-based diet, and are loaded with fiber, vitamins, minerals, and other important nutrients.

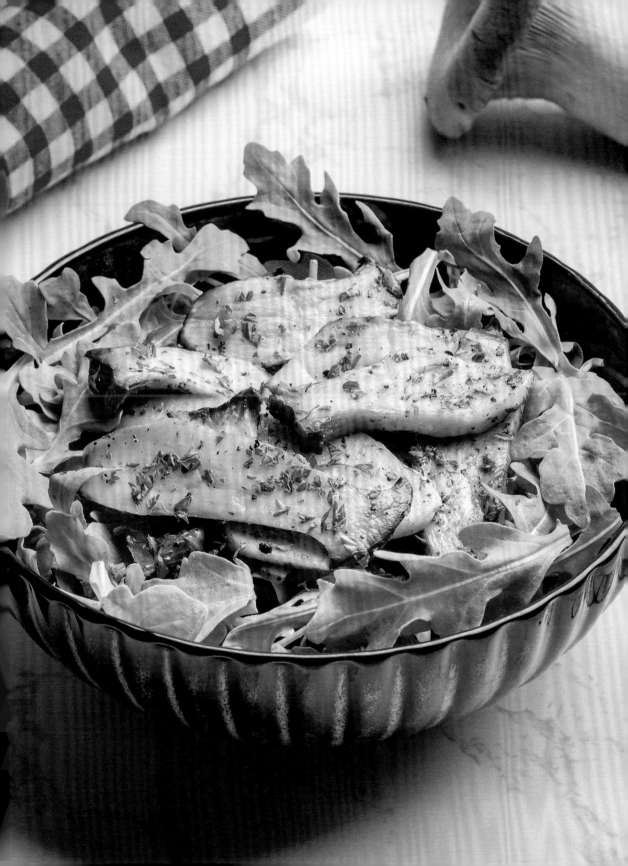

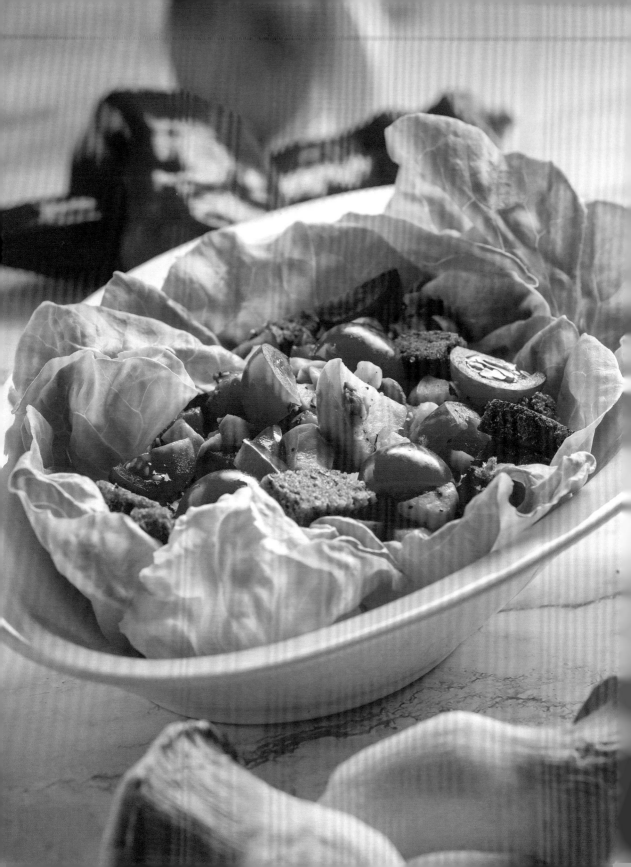

warm mushroom salad
with croutons

Oyster mushrooms have a meaty and savory flavor. They are considered a superfood because of their high nutrient content, antioxidants, and bioactive compounds. In addition, they contain beta-glucans, which boost immunity. With their hearty flavor and meaty texture, they make this salad filling. Metabolic Balance coaches in Germany shared the recipe for this salad, which is not only sweet and savory but has a satisfying, garlicky crunch from the rye bread croutons.

Makes 1 serving

4½ oz | 130 g oyster mushrooms

2 tbsp | 30 mL olive oil, divided

1 garlic clove, minced

1 slice rye bread, cut into cubes

½ red bell pepper, cut into squares

½ apple, diced

Salt and black pepper

1 tbsp | 15 mL balsamic vinegar

¼ cup | 60 mL vegetable broth

2 handfuls lamb's lettuce (mâche) or watercress

4 cherry tomatoes, halved

Clean any dirt off the mushrooms with a paper towel or the edge of a knife, but don't wash them with water. Cut the mushrooms into small pieces.

In a medium skillet, heat 1 tbsp | 15 mL of the olive oil over medium heat. Add the garlic and sauté until translucent, about 30 seconds.

Add the bread cubes and cook for 5 minutes, tossing to coat them in the garlicky oil. Transfer the croutons to a plate.

Add the mushrooms to the skillet and sauté for 3 minutes. Add the bell pepper and apple and sauté for another 2–3 minutes. Season with salt and pepper to taste.

Add the vinegar and vegetable broth and stir quickly. Remove the pan from the heat.

Put the lettuce in a bowl. Drizzle the remaining 1 tbsp | 15 mL olive oil over the lettuce and stir to coat. Arrange the lettuce on a plate and top with the mushroom mixture, garlic croutons, and tomatoes.

Special acknowledgment to Silvia Bürkle in Germany for this recipe.

SALADS

fresh **salmon salad**

Adding varied textures to dishes can make all the difference between a boring meal and an exciting one that you truly enjoy. This recipe, which comes from Metabolic Balance coaches in the UK, combines the ease of canned salmon with the texture of fresh vegetables. The cucumber gives this salmon salad a bit of crunch. Using avocado instead of mayonnaise for creaminess increases the caloric density of this salad with good fats and less sugar. Just add a sprinkle of fresh dill and serve it on a bed of lettuce for a flavorful and satisfying lunch.

Makes 1 serving

½ avocado

5 oz | 140 g can salmon, drained

6 cherry tomatoes, halved

2 tbsp | 28 g finely chopped cucumber

Salt and black pepper

Drizzle balsamic vinegar

1 dill sprig, finely chopped (optional)

In a bowl, mash the avocado. Add the salmon, flaking it apart. Add the tomatoes and cucumber and mix until creamy. Season with salt and pepper to taste and add a drizzle of vinegar. Top with a sprinkle of dill, if desired.

The Power of Protein

Proteins do most of the work in the cell and are required for the structure, function, and regulation of the body's tissues and organs. To lose weight and then maintain a healthy weight, lean muscle mass must be supported by a sufficient amount of protein.

The best sources of protein are seafood, poultry, eggs, yogurt, lean beef, milk, cheese, nuts, and seeds. Protein sources like beans, nuts, fish, and poultry are considered healthier options than red meat and full-fat dairy, which have been linked to increased risks of heart disease. However, all Metabolic Balance plans are created based on each individual's blood values and personal health history and may include many different types of protein.

Special acknowledgment to Gloria Parfitt in the United Kingdom for this recipe.

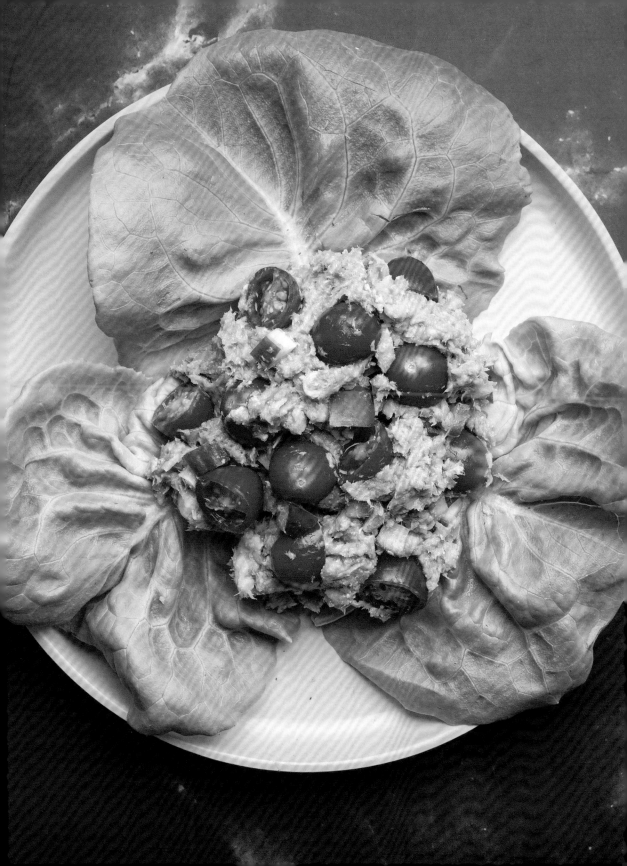

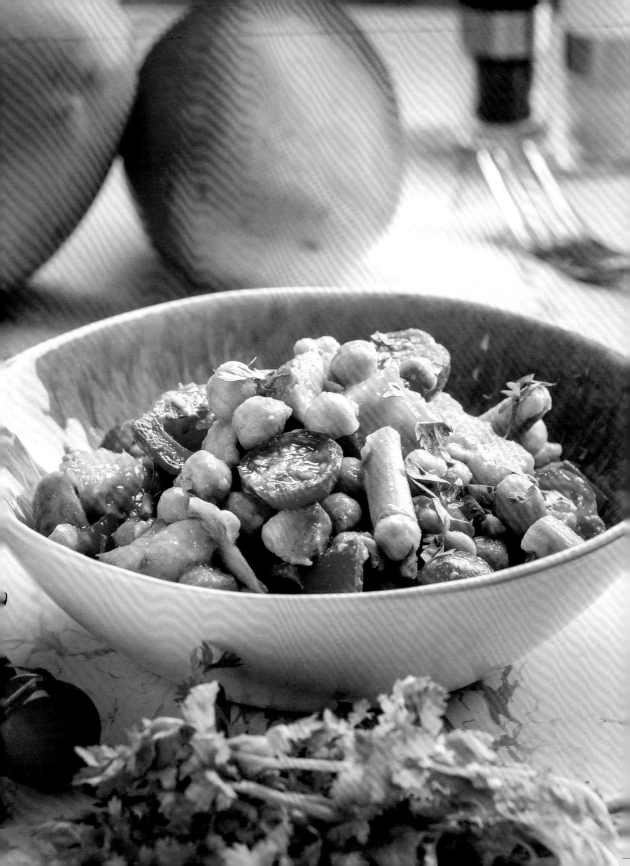

tropical chickpea and mango salad

I fell in love with mango in the Caribbean islands and spent a lot of time experimenting with it when I returned home. Because Metabolic Balance meals almost always feature a fruit (see Make It a Meal on page 30), I thought I'd try mango with chickpeas. This combination of ingredients surprised me and became one of my all-time favorite dishes. I often tell my clients to prepare this dish in the morning with frozen mango and set it aside for lunch. It's still cool and refreshing and the flavors have time to meld. I suggest using the best quality balsamic vinegar you can find as it makes all the difference.

Makes 1 serving

1 cup | 170 g canned chickpeas, drained and rinsed

1 cup | 128 g cubed mango (fresh or thawed frozen)

½ avocado, cubed

3–4 cherry tomatoes, halved

1 spring onion or green onion, sliced on the diagonal

2 tbsp | 30 mL olive oil

1 tbsp | 15 mL balsamic vinegar

1 tbsp finely chopped fresh cilantro

¼ tsp ground cumin

In a bowl, toss together the chickpeas, mango, avocado, tomatoes, and spring onion. Add the oil, vinegar, cilantro, and cumin and stir to combine.

About the Ingredient: Chickpeas

Chickpeas, a.k.a. garbanzo beans, are the most widely consumed legume in the world. They are rich in dietary fiber, which makes them valuable for heart and digestive health. Their soluble fiber content also makes them an excellent food for maintaining healthy blood sugar levels.

green papaya salad
with shrimp

thailand

Who says that a weight loss program has to be dull or tasteless? This dish, which comes to us from the Metabolic Balance coaches in Thailand, is the epitome of a perfect summer salad. Raw papaya contains an enzyme called papain that helps in the digestion of proteins. Green (unripe) papaya has a fresh, bright flavor that tantalizes the palate.

Makes 1 serving

4½ oz | 130 g large shrimp

2 tsp | 10 mL coconut oil

Salt and black pepper

2 garlic cloves

2 Thai red chiles

2 tbsp | 30 mL
fresh lime juice

1 tbsp | 15 mL fish sauce

2 tsp | 10 mL
tamarind juice

1 cup | 150 g julienned
green papaya

3 cherry tomatoes,
quartered

2 tbsp finely chopped
fresh cilantro

Remove the shrimp heads and peel, leaving the tails intact. Use a sharp knife to slit each shrimp down the back and remove the vein.

In a small skillet, heat the oil over medium heat. Add the shrimp, season with salt and pepper to taste, and sauté until just cooked through, about 2 minutes. Take care not to overcook. Set the shrimp aside.

In a mortar and pestle, pound the garlic and chiles until there are no big pieces. (Alternatively, mince the garlic and chiles with a kitchen knife on a cutting board until they form a paste, then transfer to a small bowl.) Add the lime juice, fish sauce, and tamarind juice and mix well.

In a large bowl, combine the papaya and tomatoes. Add the garlic and chile dressing and the cilantro and mix well. Toss in the shrimp.

About the Ingredient: Papaya

Papayas are on Metabolic Balance meal plans in every country. They cleanse, soothe the digestive tract, and alleviate flatulence. They are also high in antioxidants, including vitamins A, D, and E. When consumed regularly, these antioxidants can help reduce the risk of heart disease.

Special acknowledgment to Erna Hundt in Thailand for this recipe.

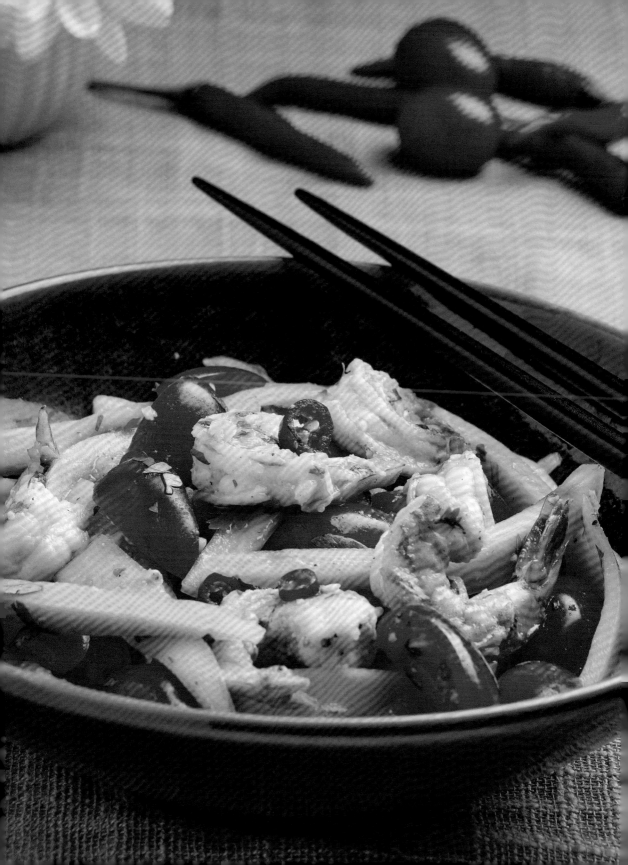

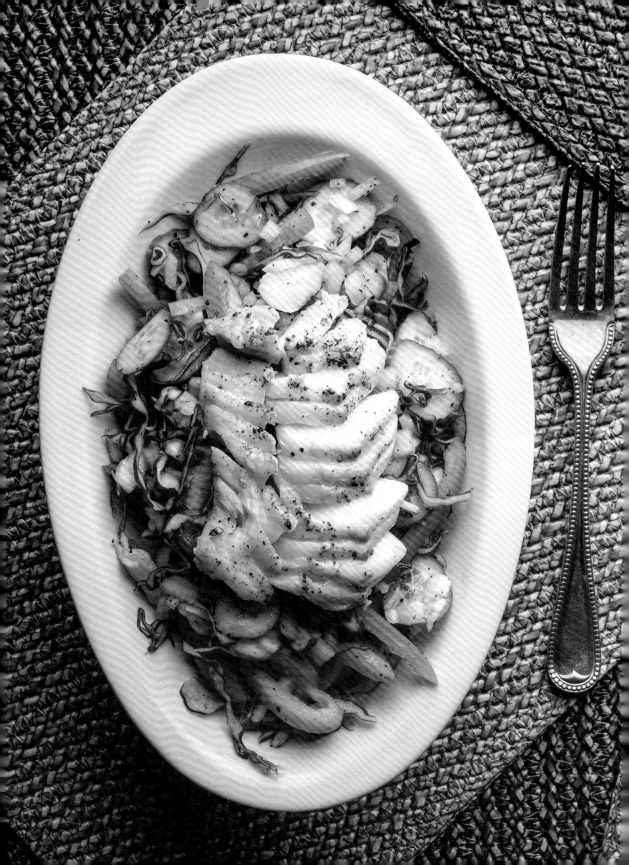

fish salad
with white onion

Previously, when I thought of a fish salad, I immediately visualized a hunk of fish on a bed of greens. This recipe from Metabolic Balance coaches in the United Arab Emirates changed my perspective. As a nutritionist, I'm always encouraging my clients to eat a rainbow of colors, and this salad more than delivers. It can be made with any white fish with firm flesh, but choose one that will grill well, such as cod, haddock, or halibut. Serve it over your favorite salad greens.

Makes 1 serving

4½ oz | 130 g white fish

½ white onion,
diced and optionally
soaked (see tip)

½ mini cucumber,
thinly sliced

¼ orange bell pepper,
thinly sliced

½ cup | 100 g
red cabbage leaves,
thinly sliced

¼ tsp ground sumac

2 tsp | 10 mL flaxseed oil

Salt

Heat a grill over high heat (or use a grill pan on the stove over high heat). Grill the fish until it is cooked through and flakes easily with a fork, 3–4 minutes per side. Cut into bite-size pieces and put in a bowl.

Add the onion, cucumber, bell pepper, cabbage, sumac, and oil and gently toss. Season with salt to taste.

TIP: When a finished dish features raw onion, like this salad does, soaking it before using it in the recipe will help to mellow its pungency. Put the diced or sliced onion in a small bowl, cover with water, and set aside to soak for at least 5 minutes while you're preparing everything else, then drain well before adding it to the recipe.

Special acknowledgment to Artemis Spörri in the United Arab Emirates for this recipe.

SALADS

incredible
mediterranean salad

greece

If you've ever traveled to Greece, hopefully you enjoyed a fresh salad while there. We have all heard that the Mediterranean diet is the healthiest as it focuses on fresh fish, fruits, vegetables, nuts, and whole grains and is very low in unhealthy fats and sugars. Not to mention, a Mediterranean meal is usually extremely colorful, and the combination of flavors explodes in your mouth. The Metabolic Balance coaches in Greece shared this authentic recipe.

Makes 1 serving

1 Roma tomato, chopped

¼ green bell pepper, chopped

¼ cucumber, chopped

¼ red onion, chopped

½ cup | 80 g crumbled or cubed feta cheese

5 pitted olives, cut in half

2 tbsp | 30 mL olive oil

Juice of ½ lemon

½ tsp fresh basil

Toss the tomato, bell pepper, cucumber, and onion together in a bowl. Add the feta and olives. Drizzle with the oil and lemon juice, sprinkle the basil on top, and toss again.

About the Ingredient: Cucumber

Cucumbers have a reputation as the best kidney cleanser. They are a diuretic, prevent bloating due to water retention, and help wash the kidneys and bladder of debris and stones.

Special acknowledgment to Konstantina Karas in Greece for this recipe.

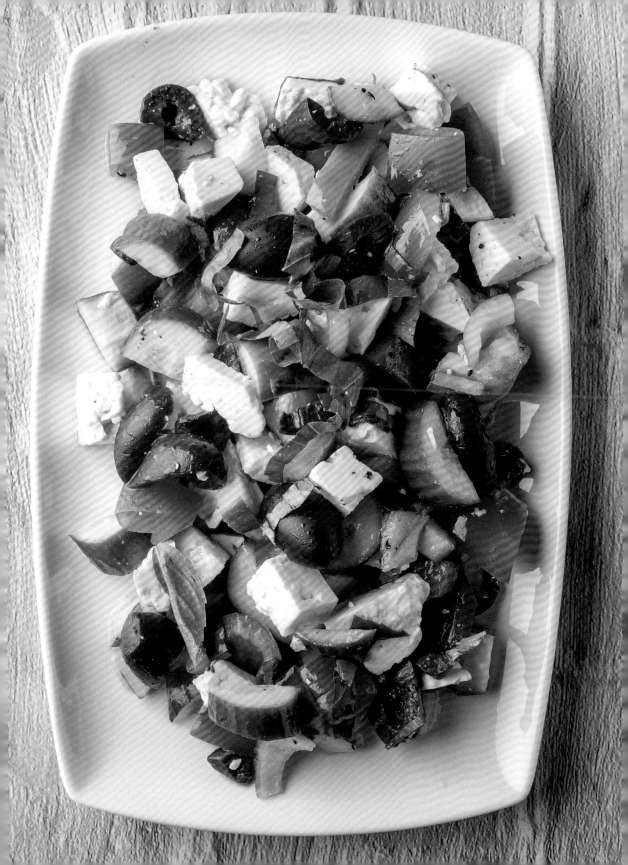

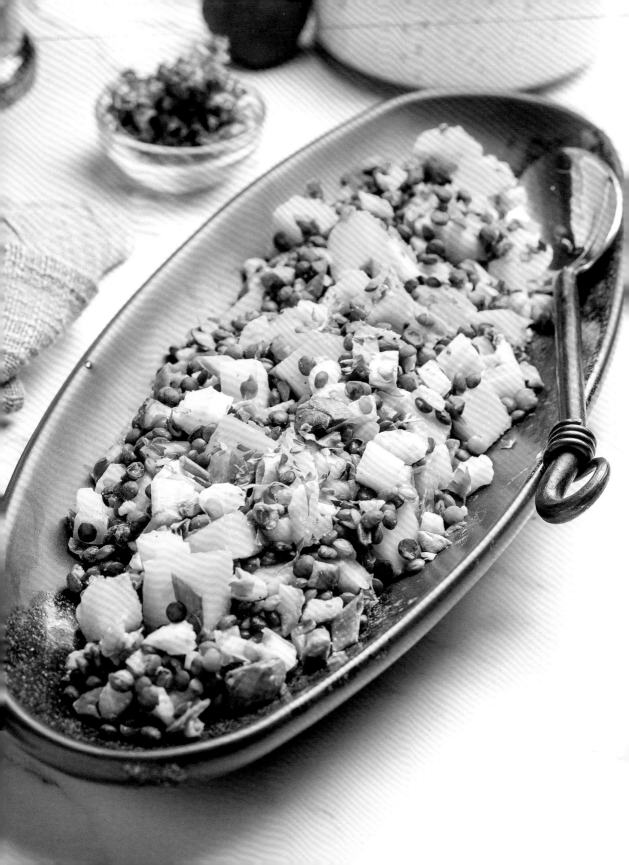

brazilian **lentil salad**

brazil

Unlike other legumes, lentils don't need to be soaked before cooking, making them a quick and easy way to add plant-based protein to your diet. A long time ago, a friend told me that cutting your green onions on the diagonal increases the exposed surface area, which increases their flavor. Give that method a try when you make this salad for a very refreshing taste. The hint of ginger also gives it zing! Thank you to Brazil's Metabolic Balance coaches for this hearty dish.

Makes 1 serving

⅓ cup | 80 g brown or black lentils, rinsed

1¼ cups | 300 mL water

1 (1-in | 2.5-cm) piece fresh ginger, grated

1 tbsp | 15 mL apple cider vinegar

½ tsp | 2.5 mL Dijon mustard

1 tsp vegetable broth powder

Salt and black pepper

1 celery rib, thinly sliced

2 green onions, sliced on the diagonal

2 cremini mushrooms, thinly sliced

1 cup | 125 g cubed mango

1 tbsp chopped fresh parsley

Combine the lentils and water in a small saucepan and bring to a boil. Reduce the heat to a simmer, cover the pan, and cook until the lentils are tender but not mushy, about 18 minutes.

Drain the lentils, if needed. In a medium bowl, mix together the ginger, vinegar, mustard, and vegetable broth powder. Season with salt and pepper to taste. Toss in the cooked lentils, celery, green onions, mushrooms, and mango. Stir to combine well.

Cover the bowl and allow the salad to marinate for 1 hour at room temperature. Top with the parsley.

Special acknowledgment to Melissa Pancini in Brazil for this recipe.

SALADS

citrus and herb salad
for a crowd

treat meal

When I ran marathons, our group of 8 hosted dinner parties at which we consumed a lot of delicious food. Like running, our dinner parties nearly became a competition too. My dear friend Sara made this salad one night, and it's been a regular item on my family's meal plan ever since. It can serve as an accompaniment to any dinner dish but can also stand alone at lunch. You will want to lick the bowl.

Makes 12 servings

Dressing

1 (3½-oz | 100-mL) jar capers, drained

Juice of 2 oranges

¾ cup | 180 mL olive oil

2 tbsp | 30 mL balsamic vinegar

2 tbsp | 30 mL white wine vinegar

1 tbsp | 15 mL honey-Dijon mustard

Salt and black pepper

Salad

1 head romaine lettuce, roughly chopped

1 head Bibb lettuce, roughly chopped

1 head green leaf lettuce, roughly chopped

1 bunch arugula, roughly chopped

1 bunch watercress, roughly chopped

1 bunch cilantro, roughly chopped

1 bunch basil, roughly chopped

¾ cup | 60 g grated Asiago cheese

½ cup | 125 g slivered almonds, toasted

1 navel orange, segmented and cut into bite-size pieces

1 pint | 345 g blueberries (optional)

To make the dressing, combine all the ingredients in a jar and shake well.

To make the salad, combine all the greens and herbs in a large bowl.

Pour in the dressing and toss well. Garnish with the cheese, almonds, orange pieces, and blueberries, if using.

TIP: If an orange isn't available, use only the blueberries.

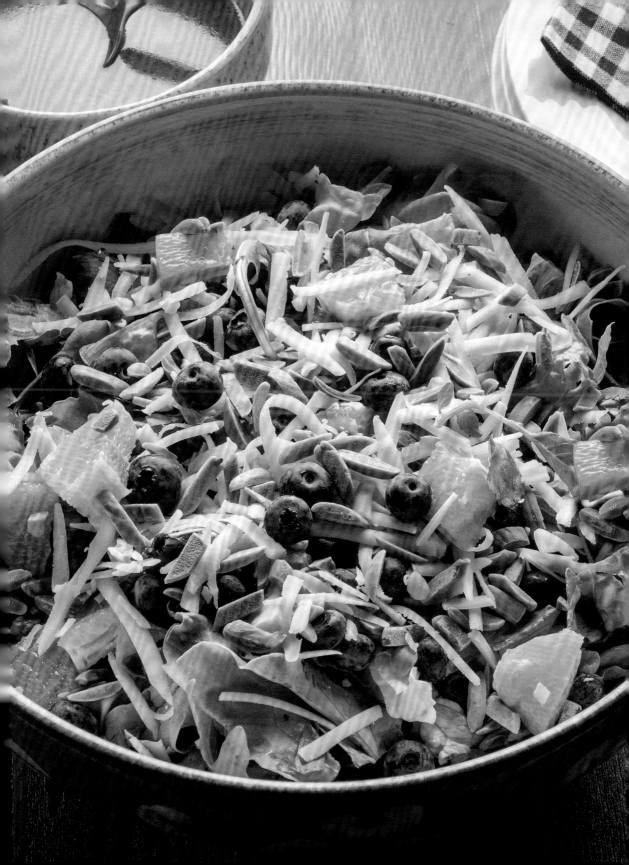

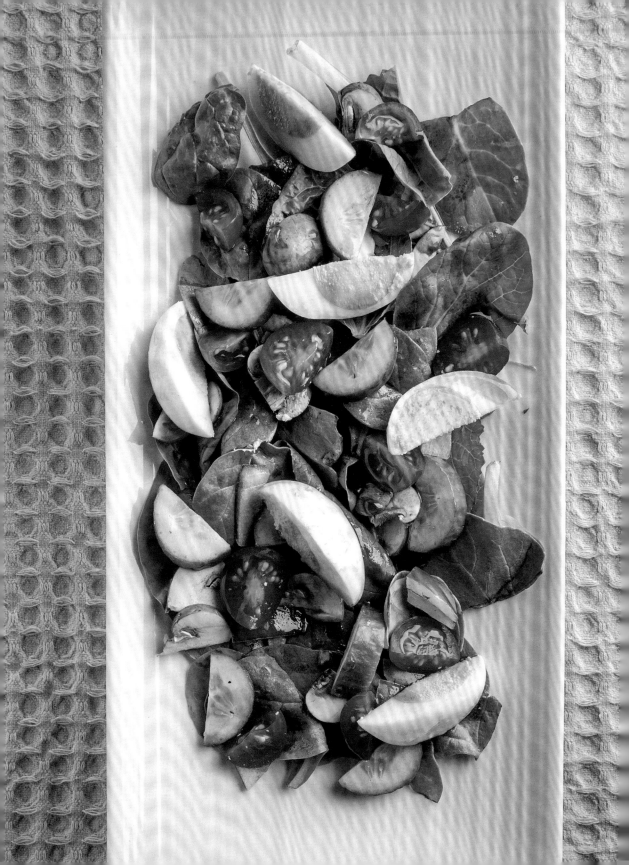

power-packed
spinach and egg salad

Spinach is known as one of the world's healthiest foods. It's an excellent plant-based source of iron, and this delicious salad provides a powerful punch. Spinach is rich in many nutrients, with at least 13 different flavonoid phytonutrients, including beta-carotene, lutein, and quercetin, which function as antioxidants. And with the eggs, this dish is also a perfect protein source.

Makes 1 serving

2 large eggs

1 tbsp | 15 mL olive oil

1 tsp | 5 mL
balsamic vinegar

¼ tsp | 1.25 mL
Dijon mustard

Salt and black pepper

1 handful baby spinach

4 cherry tomatoes,
quartered

2 button mushrooms,
thinly sliced

¼ mini cucumber,
thinly sliced

⅛ medium red onion,
thinly sliced

Fill a saucepan with enough water to cover 2 eggs. Bring to a boil, then carefully add the eggs to the saucepan. Reduce the heat to low and simmer for 10 minutes.

Pour out the hot water and run cold water over the eggs to stop them from further cooking. Allow them to cool. Peel and slice the eggs into quarters.

Meanwhile, in a small bowl, whisk together the oil, vinegar, mustard, and salt and pepper to taste. Arrange the spinach, tomatoes, mushrooms, cucumber, and onion on a plate and top with the eggs.

Drizzle the dressing over the salad.

TIP: If you are missing the crunch of bacon bits on your salad, crumble up a rye cracker and sprinkle it on top to add another layer of texture.

cannellini beans
with tomato and sage

I never knew Tuscan white beans could taste so good! For years, my very busy mother cooked them for our family of eleven. She soaked and cooked them, added no flavor, and unceremoniously put them on our plates. That was dinner. So, we ate it. What those beans needed was flavor—and this dish has lots of it, thanks to just a few simple ingredients. This hearty dish contains many nutrients and a lot of fiber while being low in fat. It is a great plant-based protein! Serve it with rye bread or crackers.

Makes 1 serving

1 tbsp | 15 mL olive oil

1 garlic clove, minced

4 fresh sage leaves, torn if large, plus more for garnish

¼ cup vegetable broth

1 cup | 170 g canned white beans, drained and rinsed

1 medium tomato, seeded and diced

Salt and black pepper

Heat the oil in a small saucepan over medium heat. Add the garlic and sage and sauté until the garlic is lightly golden, about 1 minute. Add the vegetable broth and beans and stir. Simmer for 20 minutes, stirring occasionally to blend the flavors. Add the tomato during the last 2–3 minutes of cooking to heat. Season with salt and pepper to taste. Garnish with sage, if desired.

6 tips to reduce inflammation in the body:

- Lose excess weight
- Keep blood sugar balanced
- Reduce or manage stress
- Supplement with vitamin D
- Exercise regularly
- Keep hormones balanced

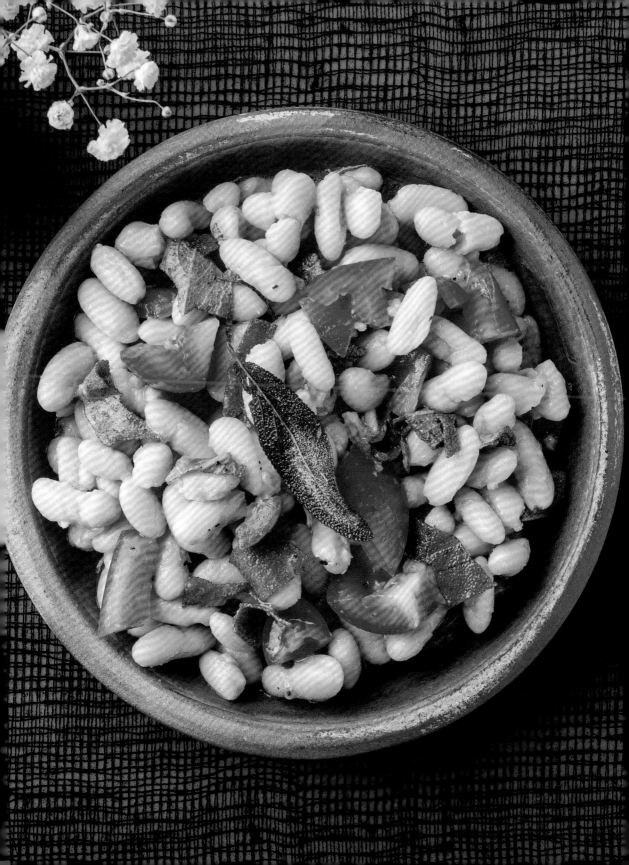

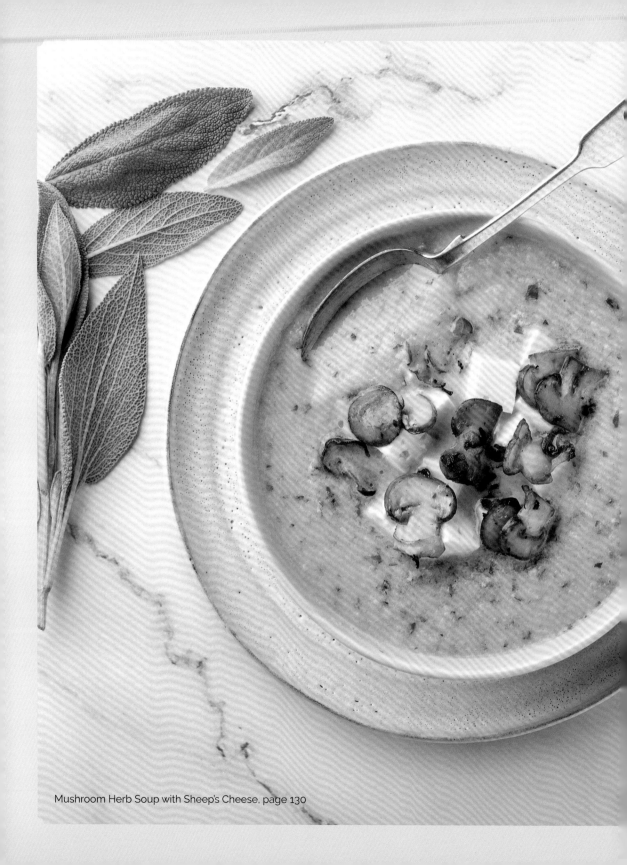

Mushroom Herb Soup with Sheep's Cheese, page 130

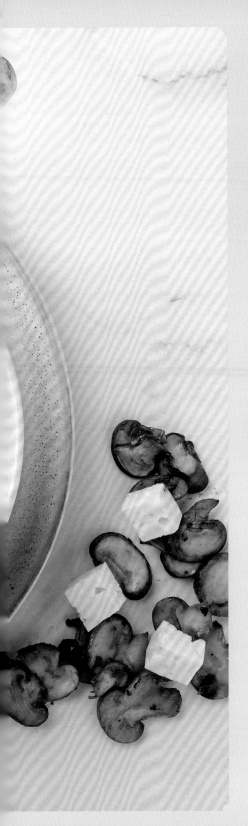

soups

The aroma of soup cooking on the stove always makes me feel warm and fuzzy on the inside as it reminds me of my childhood. Soups were staple meals in our home, and they are great comfort foods in cultures around the world. With these easy, flavorful, vegetable-forward recipes, they can also be nutrient-dense components of your diet! Soups are delicious and inexpensive, they freeze well, and they can help keep you hydrated.

cabbage soup
with smoked tofu

This soup is the definition of warm and cozy, but it is not heavy. And despite the long ingredient list, this is a very quick dish to prepare. If you think cabbage and tofu sound boring, think again! The curry, cumin, and cilantro help bring out the cabbage's natural sweetness.

Makes 1 serving

½ onion,
cut into small dice

2 tbsp | 30 mL water

¼ tsp curry powder

¼ tsp cumin seeds

1 garlic clove, minced

1½ cups | 355 mL
vegetable broth or water

¾ cup | 45 g shredded
white cabbage

½ carrot,
cut into small dice

1 (1-in | 2.5-cm) piece
fresh ginger, minced

2½ oz | 70 g smoked tofu,
cubed

1 tbsp chopped fresh
cilantro leaves,
plus more for garnish

Salt and black pepper

In a medium saucepan, combine the onion and water. Cover and steam over medium-low heat for 2 minutes.

Season with the curry powder, cumin, and garlic and stir to coat the onion. Add the broth, cabbage, carrot, and ginger, increase the heat to medium, and simmer, uncovered, until the vegetables are soft, about 15 minutes.

Add the tofu and cilantro and cook for 5 minutes. Season with salt and pepper to taste.

Garnish with cilantro, if desired.

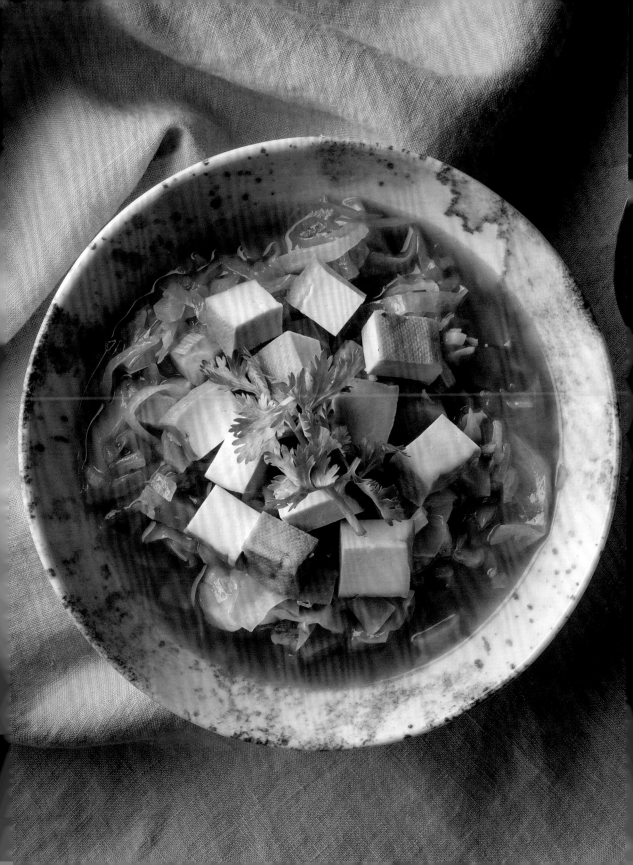

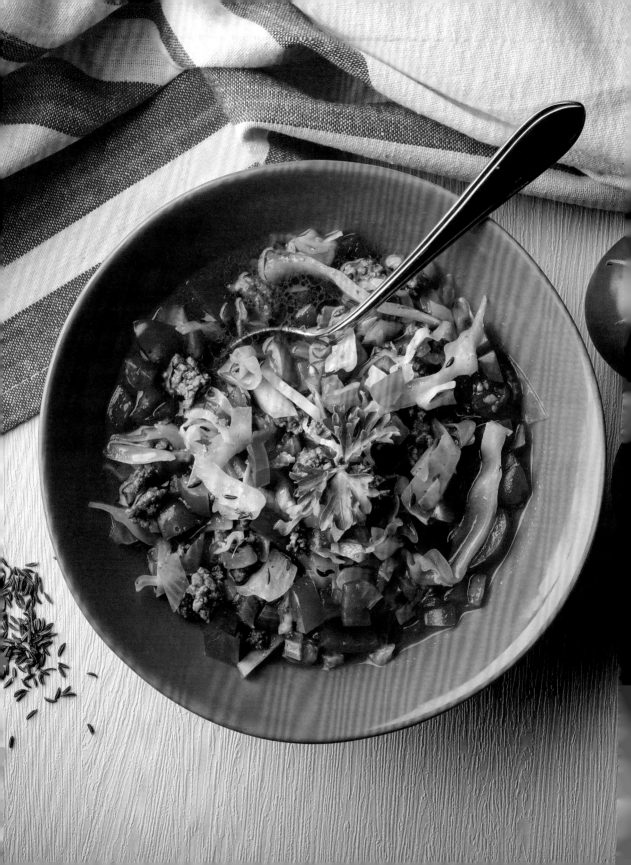

cabbage roll soup
with beef

This hearty, flavorful soup brings back nostalgic memories of beef-stuffed cabbage rolls, without all the time-consuming work of steaming, stuffing, and baking. Caraway seeds add a wonderful flavor to this soup.

Makes 1 serving

½ onion, diced

1 celery rib, diced

4½ oz | 130 g beef tenderloin, ground (see page 191)

1 garlic clove, minced

¼ tsp dried parsley

¼ tsp caraway seeds

1 cup | 60 g shredded white cabbage

1 tomato, diced

1 cup | 240 mL vegetable broth

Salt and black pepper

Fresh parsley leaves, for garnish (optional)

In a medium saucepan, cook the onion and celery over medium-high heat for 2 minutes, stirring constantly to prevent burning.

Add the ground beef tenderloin, garlic, parsley, and caraway seeds and cook, stirring, for another 2 minutes.

Add the cabbage, tomato, and broth, turn the heat down to medium, and simmer for 15 minutes, or until the beef is cooked through and the cabbage is soft. Season with salt and pepper. Garnish with fresh parsley, if desired.

Can I use chicken or beef broth for cooking while on the Metabolic Balance program?

No chicken or beef (or other protein-containing) broth is allowed on the program. It is recommended that you eat only 1 protein at each meal, and get an optimum amount of it according to your plan. Eating two different types of proteins at a time leads to over-acidification (see Metabolic Balance Rule #5, page 60), which makes it difficult to lose weight. Veggie broth is packed with minerals like calcium and magnesium and vitamins like A, C, E, and K, and it's also low in calories and high in fiber.

velvety chicken soup

Most of us walk by the parsnips in the grocery aisle because we don't know what to do with them. The parsnips in this smooth, pureed soup add a surprising sweetness and a creamy texture. Parsnips enhance anti-inflammatory properties, contain healthy fiber, and are high in vitamin C. Nutritious and delicious!

Makes 1 serving

4½ oz | 130 g boneless, skinless chicken (or turkey) breast

½ medium carrot, cut into medium dice

½ parsnip (big end), cut into medium dice

¼ orange bell pepper, cut into medium dice

1 garlic clove, chopped

1¼ cups | 300 mL vegetable broth

¼ tsp paprika

Salt and black pepper

Finely chopped fresh parsley, for garnish

Cut the chicken into cubes. In a medium saucepan, combine the chicken, carrot, parsnip, bell pepper, garlic, broth, paprika, and salt and pepper to taste. Cook over medium-low heat for 30–40 minutes, until the chicken is cooked through and the vegetables are tender.

Using an immersion blender, blend the soup until smooth, or transfer the chicken and vegetables plus a little broth to a blender or food processor and puree. Then return the puree to the pot and stir.

Check the seasoning and adjust as needed. Serve garnished with parsley.

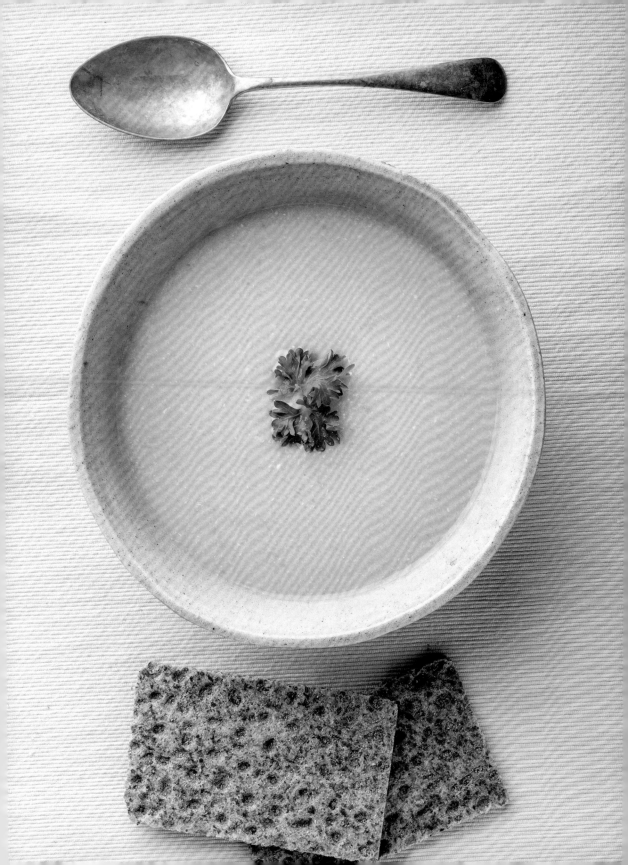

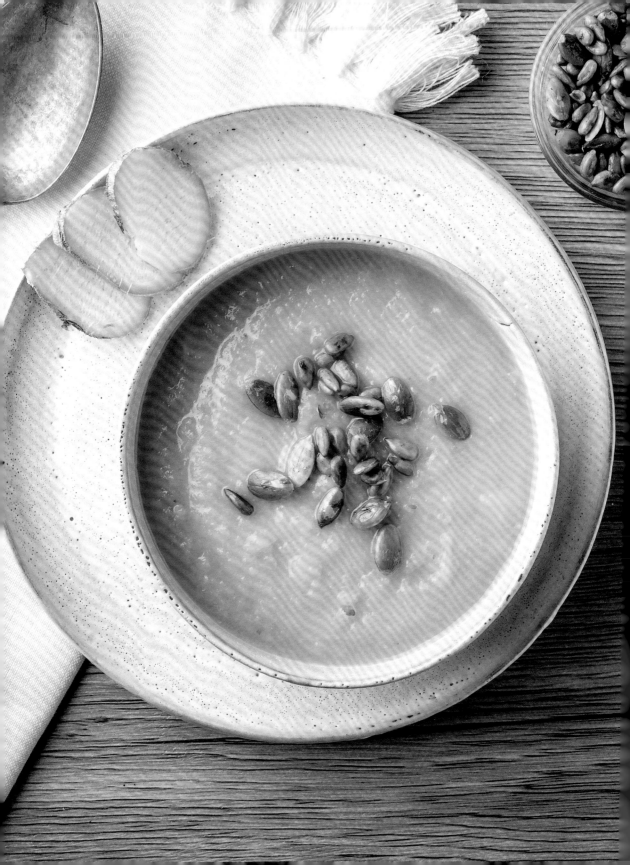

pumpkin ginger soup

This soup makes me feel like I'm in a fine restaurant with its tremendous eye appeal, yet it takes only minutes to make. The seeds add an extra crunch, like a crouton.

Makes 1 serving

2 tbsp | 20 g
pumpkin seeds

2 tbsp | 20 g
sunflower seeds

1 cup | 115 g roughly
chopped pumpkin or
butternut squash

⅓ onion, diced

1 garlic clove, minced

½ red chile pepper,
seeded and thinly sliced

1 (1-in | 2.5-cm) piece
fresh ginger,
finely chopped

Leaves from 1 rosemary
sprig, finely chopped

1¼ cups | 300 mL
vegetable broth

Salt and black pepper

Heat a nonstick skillet over medium-high heat. Add the pumpkin seeds and sunflower seeds and toast, stirring frequently, for 2–3 minutes. Transfer the seeds to a plate and set aside.

In a medium saucepan, combine the pumpkin, onion, garlic, chile, ginger, and rosemary. Add the broth and cook over medium-low heat until the pumpkin is soft, about 15 minutes.

Using an immersion blender, blend the soup until smooth, or transfer the soup to a blender or food processor and puree.

Season with salt and pepper to taste. Add the toasted pumpkin seeds and sunflower seeds to the soup, reserving a few for a garnish.

Have Fun!

When people go on a weight loss plan, they often think the foods will be boring. With Metabolic Balance, that's simply not the case. Those who are committed to this way of life, and want to maintain a balanced weight and healthy metabolism, are more successful due to the variety of foods allowed. Recipe experimentation is fun and keeps everyone motivated.

pumpkin soup
with shiitakes

Vegetables with an orange hue are loaded with beta-carotene, an important nutrient for eye and skin health. Pumpkin is a carbohydrate and tastes great when roasted. Sautéing the mushrooms without oil helps reset your metabolism so you can lose weight more effectively.

Makes 1 serving

5 oz | 145 g
shiitake mushrooms

1 cup | 115 g
diced pumpkin

½ carrot, diced

1 tbsp diced onion

1 (1-in | 2.5-cm) piece
fresh ginger, minced

2 tbsp | 30 mL water

1 tsp curry powder

1 cup | 240 mL
vegetable broth

2 tbsp | 30 mL
fresh lemon juice

Salt and black pepper

Clean any dirt off the mushrooms with a paper towel or the edge of a knife, but don't wash them with water. Cut the mushrooms into thin slices.

In a medium saucepan, combine the pumpkin, carrot, onion, ginger, and water. Steam over medium heat for about 3 minutes, or until the pumpkin and carrot are soft but still firm.

Add the curry powder and broth and cook for 20 minutes.

Meanwhile, heat a small skillet over medium heat and sauté the mushrooms for 2–4 minutes, stirring frequently, until softened. Set aside.

Using an immersion blender, blend the soup until smooth, or transfer the soup to a blender or food processor and puree, then return the soup to the pan.

Add the lemon juice and season with salt and pepper to taste. Cook over low heat for 5 minutes.

Top the soup with the mushrooms and serve.

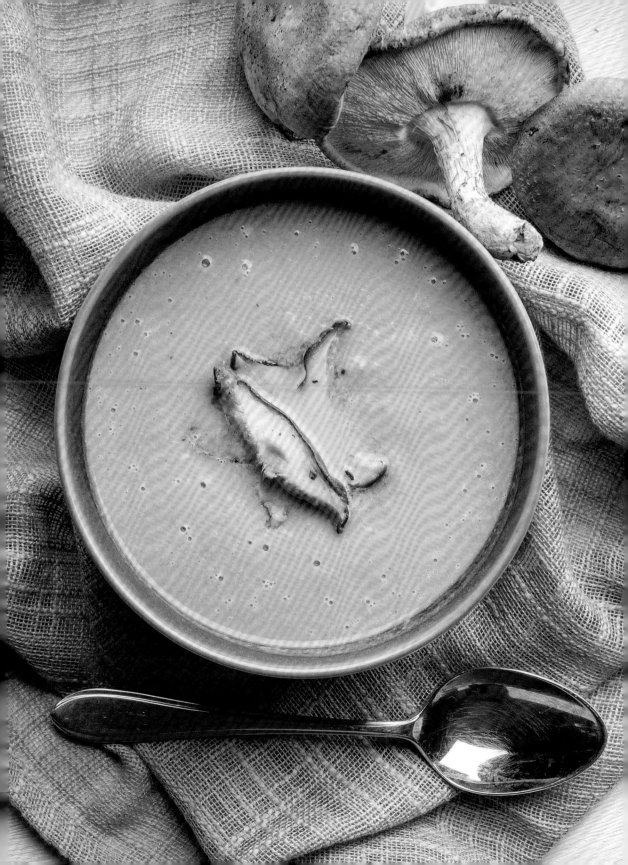

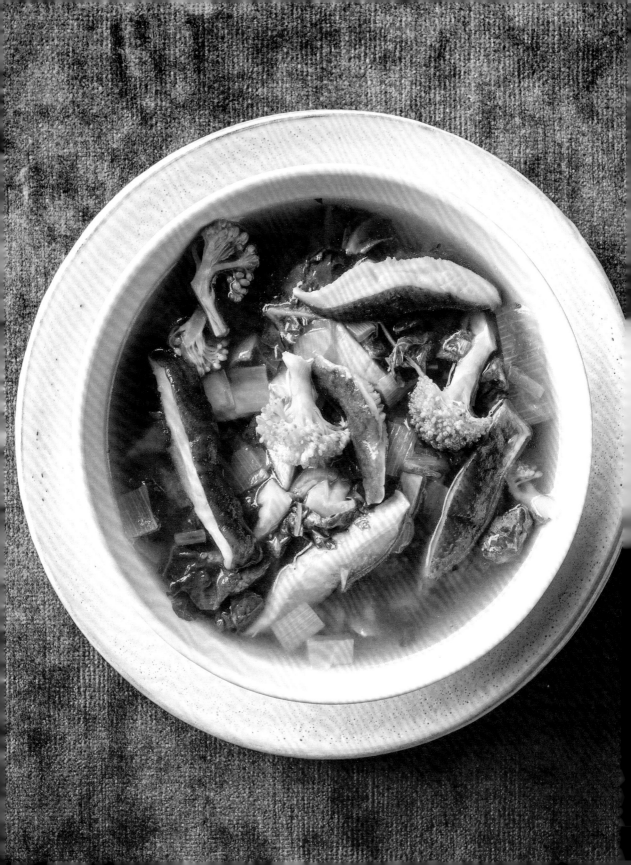

rich shiitake mushroom soup

In traditional Chinese medicine, shiitake mushrooms are believed to improve one's life energy, or chi. They contain compounds that can help lower your cholesterol and stimulate your immune system. This vegetarian soup tastes rich thanks to those protein-rich mushrooms.

Makes 1 serving

5 oz | 145 g
shiitake mushrooms

1⅓ cups | 315 mL
vegetable broth

1 cup | 70 g chopped
bok choy

¾ cup | 38 g
chopped leek

½ cup | 35 g
broccoli florets

Pinch ground cumin

Salt and black pepper

Chopped fresh cilantro
leaves, for garnish
(optional)

½ tsp black sesame
seeds, for garnish
(optional)

Clean any dirt off the mushrooms with a paper towel or the edge of a knife, but don't wash them with water. Cut the mushrooms into thin slices.

Combine the mushrooms and broth in a medium saucepan and cook over medium heat for 3 minutes. Add the bok choy, leek, and broccoli and simmer until the broccoli is softened, about 12 minutes.

Add the cumin and season with salt and pepper to taste. If desired, add the cilantro leaves and black sesame seeds, for garnish.

mushroom herb soup
with sheep's cheese

germany

Smooth and sweet, this soup from Metabolic Balance coaches in Germany gets extra protein from the tasty, creamy sheep's cheese. As many people have intolerance to cow's milk, sheep's (or goat feta) cheese is a great alternative. The sautéed mushrooms add a lovely texture to this soup and the herbs give it a rich flavor.

Makes 1 serving

2 tbsp | 30 mL olive oil, divided

½ cup | 50 g diced red onion

1 garlic clove, minced

1 cup | 135 g chopped parsnip

1 cup | 240 mL vegetable broth

2 cremini or button mushrooms, thinly sliced

1 tbsp finely chopped fresh sage, basil, and/or parsley

Salt and black pepper

½ cup | 80 g crumbled or cubed sheep's or goat feta cheese

Heat 1 tbsp | 15 mL of the oil in a small saucepan over medium heat. Add the onion and garlic and sauté for 2 minutes. Add the parsnip and stir to coat with the oil. Pour in the broth and bring to a boil.

Reduce the heat to medium-low and simmer for about 15 minutes, or until the parsnip is soft.

Meanwhile, heat the remaining 1 tbsp | 15 mL oil in a small skillet over medium heat. Add the mushrooms and sauté for 5 minutes, then set aside.

Using an immersion blender, blend the soup until smooth, or transfer the soup to a blender or food processor and puree, then return the soup to the pan.

Add the mushrooms and fresh herbs to the soup and stir to heat through. Season with salt and pepper to taste and top with the cheese.

Pictured on page 116

Special acknowledgment to Silvia Bürkle in Germany for this recipe.

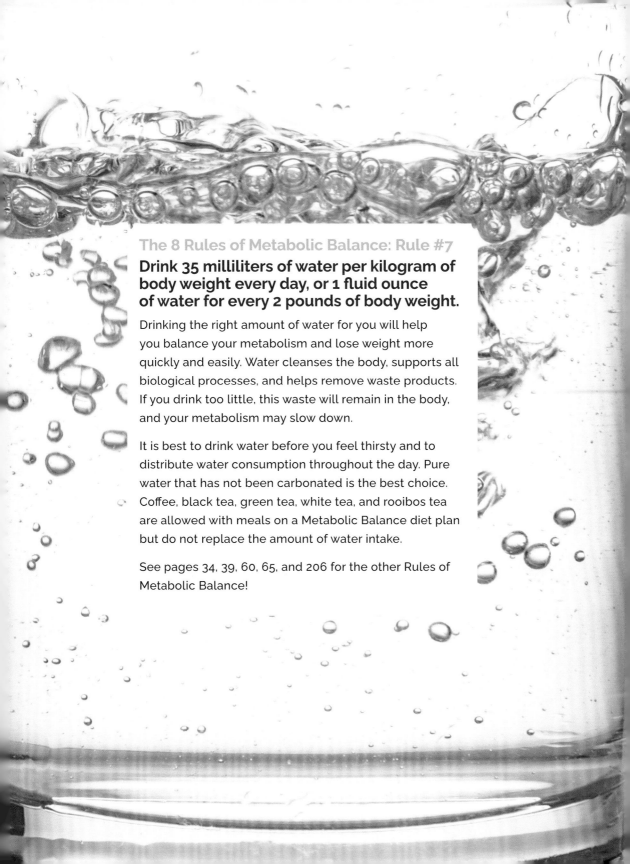

The 8 Rules of Metabolic Balance: Rule #7

Drink 35 milliliters of water per kilogram of body weight every day, or 1 fluid ounce of water for every 2 pounds of body weight.

Drinking the right amount of water for you will help you balance your metabolism and lose weight more quickly and easily. Water cleanses the body, supports all biological processes, and helps remove waste products. If you drink too little, this waste will remain in the body, and your metabolism may slow down.

It is best to drink water before you feel thirsty and to distribute water consumption throughout the day. Pure water that has not been carbonated is the best choice. Coffee, black tea, green tea, white tea, and rooibos tea are allowed with meals on a Metabolic Balance diet plan but do not replace the amount of water intake.

See pages 34, 39, 60, 65, and 206 for the other Rules of Metabolic Balance!

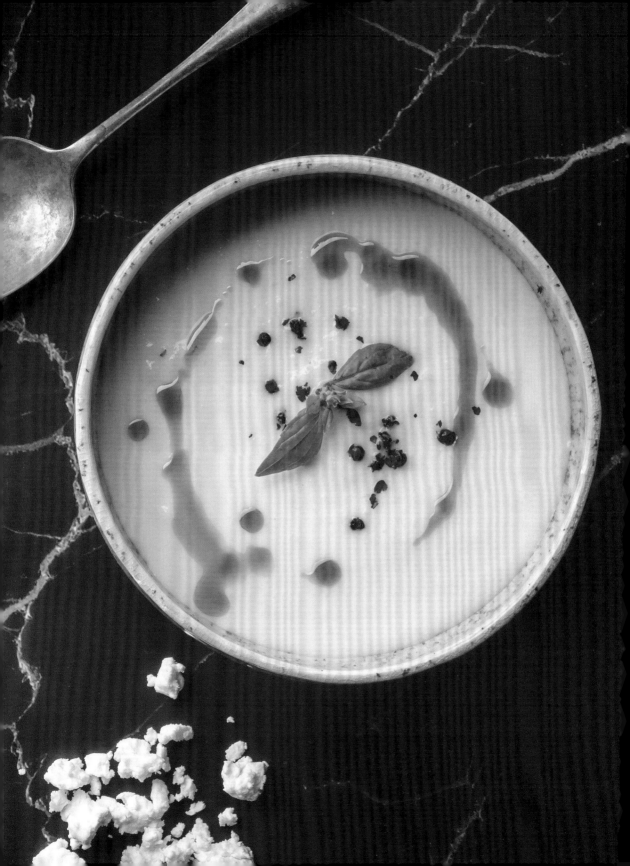

delicious
du barry cream soup

france

Transport yourself to Paris with this incredibly delicious soup from Metabolic Balance coaches in France. It is reminiscent of the creaminess of vichyssoise but uses the versatility of fresh goat cheese as a replacement for cream, and for protein. It is easy to prepare and has become a go-to soup in my household. Serve it warm with some toasted rye bread. C'est magnifique!

Makes 2 servings

½ medium cauliflower head, cored and cut into florets

1 shallot, minced

1 garlic clove, minced

2 cups | 475 mL vegetable broth

½ tsp ground nutmeg

Salt and black pepper

1 cup | 160 g crumbled goat or sheep's cheese

Thinly sliced fresh basil, for garnish

Pink or black peppercorn berries, for garnish

1 tbsp | 15 mL pumpkin seed oil, for drizzling

In a large saucepan, combine the cauliflower, shallot, garlic, and broth. Bring to a boil over medium heat.

Add the nutmeg and season with salt and pepper to taste. Cover the pan and simmer over low heat for 20 minutes, or until the cauliflower is tender (a knife blade should go through the florets very easily).

Add the cheese. Using an immersion blender, blend the soup until smooth, or transfer the soup to a blender or food processor and puree, then return the soup to the pan. Warm the soup over low heat for another 5 minutes.

Divide the soup into 2 bowls. Garnish with the basil and a few peppercorn berries and drizzle with the pumpkin seed oil.

Special acknowledgment to Laurent Causse in France for this recipe.

SOUPS

chickpea soup with mint

The slightly nutty taste of chickpeas is a good complement to the heat of the chiles and the freshness of mint in this soup—a surprising flavor combination that is reminiscent of summer at any time of the year. People tend to really like the buttery texture of chickpeas as it holds its own in dishes.

Makes 1 serving

1¼ cups | 300 mL
vegetable broth

½ cup | 50 g
cauliflower florets

8 small cherry tomatoes,
halved

¼ small red onion,
minced

1 garlic clove,
finely chopped

½ red chile pepper,
seeded and thinly sliced

1 cup | 170 g
canned chickpeas,
drained and rinsed

1 tbsp finely chopped
fresh mint

Salt and black pepper

In a small saucepan, bring the broth to a boil over medium-high heat. Add the cauliflower, tomatoes, onion, garlic, and chile. Reduce the heat to medium and simmer briskly for about 5 minutes, until the cauliflower can be pierced by a fork.

Add the chickpeas and mint, stir to combine, and season with salt and pepper to taste.

With Metabolic Balance, you can:

- Promote and maintain an improved quality of life
- Enhance your vitality and performance
- Reset your metabolism
- Fight inflammation
- Achieve and maintain a healthy weight
- Increase your resistance to personal and professional stress
- Detox your body on a cellular level
- Balance hunger hormones
- Stay fit well into your senior years

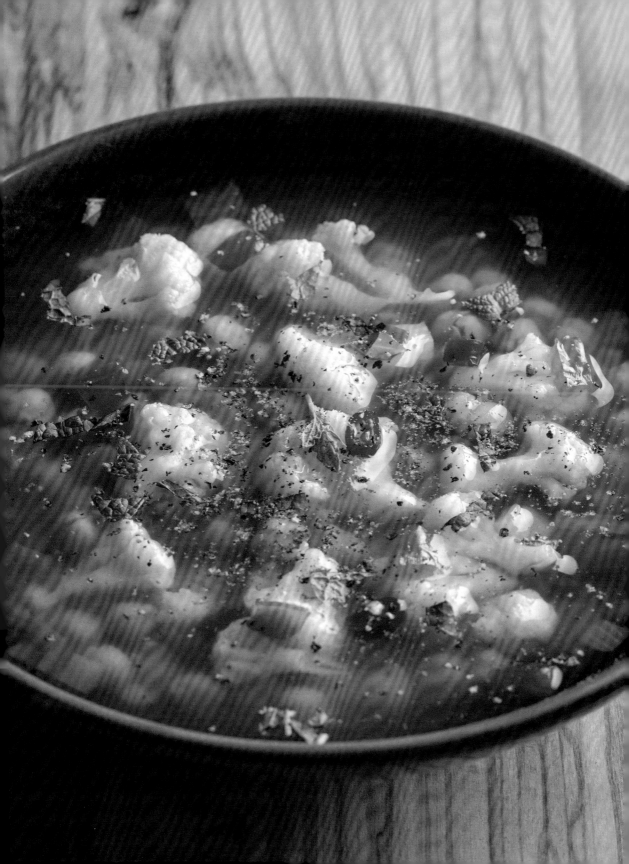

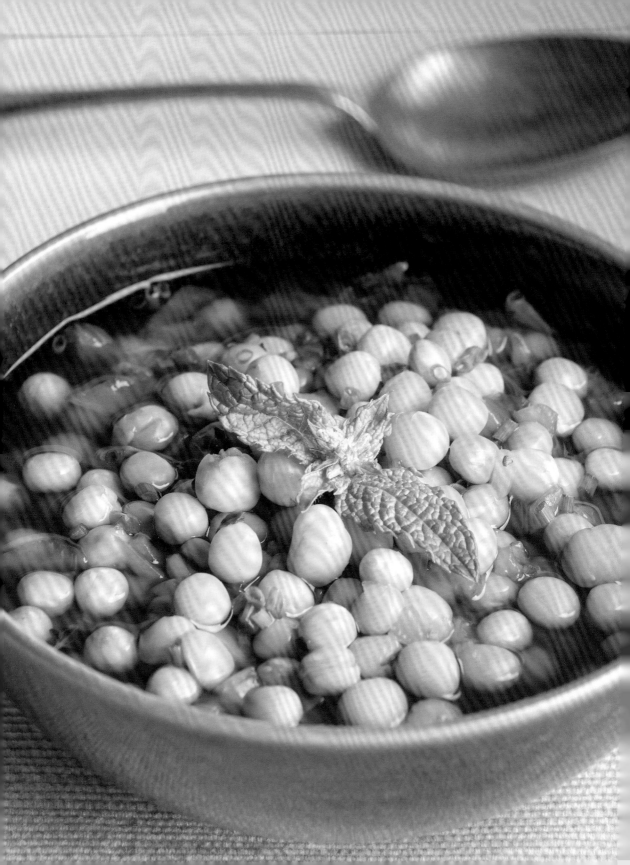

protein-packed
savory pea soup

sweden

This hearty and delicious soup is brought to us by Metabolic Balance coaches in Sweden. Peas are an important source of protein, rich in vitamins and minerals. Yellow peas are full of phytonutrients with antioxidative and anti-inflammatory properties. But peas contain lectins, which are a protective coating that defend the plant from predators in nature. By soaking and cooking, we neutralize the lectins. (Cooking time can be greatly reduced for those who like to use a pressure cooker.)

Makes 4 servings

1 cup | 225 g dried whole yellow peas

1 yellow onion, finely chopped

1 tsp dried thyme

1 tsp dried marjoram (optional), plus more for garnish

1 chive, minced

Salt and black pepper

Fresh mint leaves, for garnish (optional)

Put the peas in a large bowl and cover with plenty of water, at least 3 times the volume of the peas. Let them sit for 8–12 hours at room temperature, changing the water once or twice, if possible. Drain and rinse the peas.

In a medium pot, combine the peas, onion, and dried herbs. Add enough cold water to cover the peas. Bring to a gentle boil, then reduce the heat to a simmer. Cook for 1½–2 hours, or until the peas are tender, stirring occasionally. Add more water as desired to achieve your preferred consistency. Add the chive and stir.

Season the soup with salt and pepper to taste and garnish with mint leaves and more marjoram, if desired.

Protein Memory

People who go on restrictive diets generally lose muscle and not fat. When they stop the diet, they often have a ravenous hunger until their protein levels are returned to normal. This does not happen with the Metabolic Balance program because each meal is protein rich, which protects muscle and keeps the appetite balanced.

What foods contain protein? Poultry, eggs, meats, dairy products, fish and other seafood, nuts, seeds, some mushrooms, and legumes, including soy products or tofu.

Special acknowledgment to Susanna Rantala Ibsen in Sweden for this recipe.

SOUPS

tuscan **bean soup**

The long, cold Canadian winters make us northerners dream of Tuscany in the summer—vineyards, blue skies, sunshine, and aromatic smells. This soup is reminiscent of eating al fresco on a shaded Italian terrace. Thank you, Metabolic Balance coaches from Italy, for sending us this recipe, which uses easy, simple ingredients that are readily available year-round.

Makes 1 serving

1 tbsp | 15 mL
extra-virgin olive oil

½ small onion, chopped

6 fresh basil leaves,
finely chopped

1 celery rib, chopped

1 garlic clove, minced

1 bay leaf

1 cup | 170 g
canned white beans,
drained and rinsed

1⅓ cups | 315 mL
vegetable broth

Salt and black pepper

Heat the oil in a medium saucepan over medium heat. Add the onion, basil, celery, garlic, and bay leaf and cook for about 2 minutes, until softened. Add the beans and toss to coat with the oil. Heat through for a few minutes.

Pour in the broth, turn the heat down to medium-low, and bring to a simmer. Adjust the heat to maintain a bare simmer and cook for 10 minutes, or until the beans are just tender. Season with salt and pepper to taste.

TIP: If you prefer a creamy soup, remove the bay leaf and blend the soup with an immersion blender. It will have the creaminess of vichyssoise without any cream!

Special acknowledgment to Daniela Langellotti in Italy for this recipe.

THE METABOLIC BALANCE KITCHEN

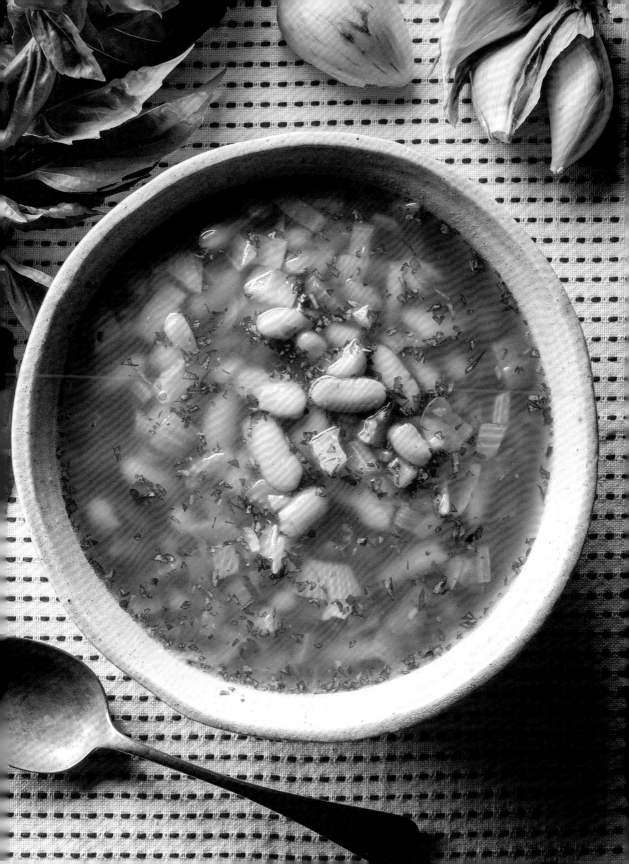

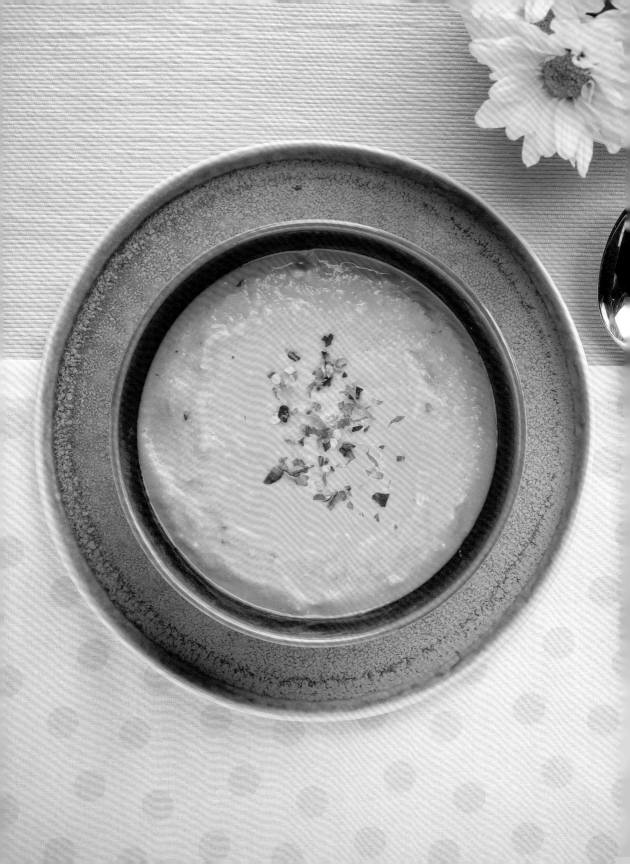

hearty **lentil soup**

turkey

This delicious lentil soup is loaded with fiber and flavor and blended smooth for a delicious velvety consistency. Many people don't realize that lentils are high in protein and are a great substitute for meat. This authentic and nourishing soup is shared by the Metabolic Balance coaches in Turkey.

Makes 4 servings

1 cup | 240 g red lentils

3 tbsp | 45 mL
olive oil

1 onion, finely chopped

1 tbsp tomato paste

3 cups | 710 mL water

1 tsp sweet paprika

1½ cups | 355 mL
vegetable broth

Salt

Chopped fresh oregano
and/or red pepper flakes,
for garnish (optional)

Rinse the lentils and set aside in a colander to drain.

Heat the oil in a large saucepan. Add the onion and sauté until tender, about 2 minutes. Stir in the tomato paste and cook for 2–3 minutes. Add the water, lentils, and paprika and stir well. Cover and cook over low heat until the lentils are fully cooked and tender, about 30 minutes.

Using an immersion blender, blend the soup until smooth, or transfer the soup to a blender or food processor and puree, then return the soup to the pan.

Add the broth and cook for 2–3 minutes, until heated through. Season with salt to taste and garnish as you like.

Special acknowledgment to Sophie Kamuran Demirtas in Turkey for this recipe.

SOUPS

tom yum hot and sour soup
with shrimp

Thailand is one of my most beloved places to visit, and Thai food is definitely a favorite. I was thrilled when the Metabolic Balance coaches from Thailand sent us this recipe. Some of the ingredients may be a little hard to find, but it's worth a search, and you may have luck buying online. This hot and sour soup has a great depth of flavor from the chile, lime, and tamarind.

Makes 4 servings

1 pound | 454 g large shrimp with shells, tails, and heads

1 tbsp | 15 mL olive oil

8 cups | 2 liters water, divided

2 tbsp | 30 mL red curry paste

2 tbsp | 30 mL tamarind puree

2 tsp ground turmeric

4–6 makrut lime leaves (see note)

1 tsp chopped red chile pepper (optional)

2 tbsp | 30 mL fish sauce

2 tbsp | 30 mL fresh lime juice

Chopped fresh cilantro leaves, for garnish

Remove the shrimp heads and shell, leaving the tails intact. Reserve the heads and shells. Use a sharp knife to slit each shrimp down the back and remove the vein.

Heat the oil in a large saucepan over medium-high heat. Add the shrimp heads and shells and cook for about 10 minutes, tossing frequently, until the heads and shells are deep orange.

Add about 1 cup | 240 mL of the water and the curry paste and bring to a simmer; cook for 5 minutes. Add the remaining water and bring to a simmer; cook for 5 more minutes.

Set a strainer over a large bowl or another pot and strain the shrimp stock. Discard the heads and shells and return the stock to the pan. Stir in the tamarind, turmeric, lime leaves, and chile, if using. Bring to a simmer and cook for 2 minutes. Add the shrimp and cook for about 3 minutes, until they turn pink.

Stir in the fish sauce and lime juice. Garnish with the cilantro.

NOTE: Makrut lime leaves, a.k.a. Thai lime leaves, are an essential ingredient in Thai cuisine. If you don't have them, you can use the zest of a lime or lemon or even some lemongrass to add a bright citrus flavor to this dish.

Special acknowledgment to Erna Hundt in Thailand for this recipe.

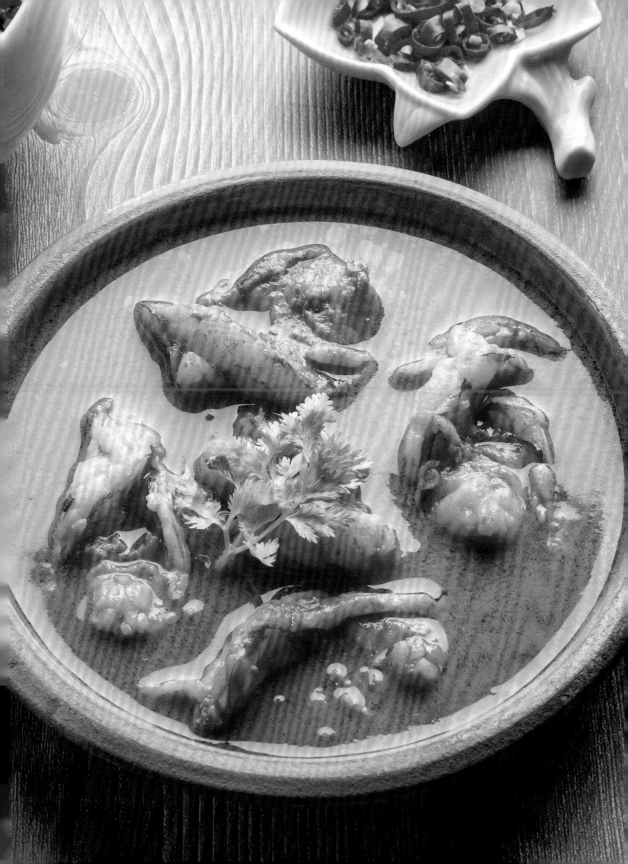

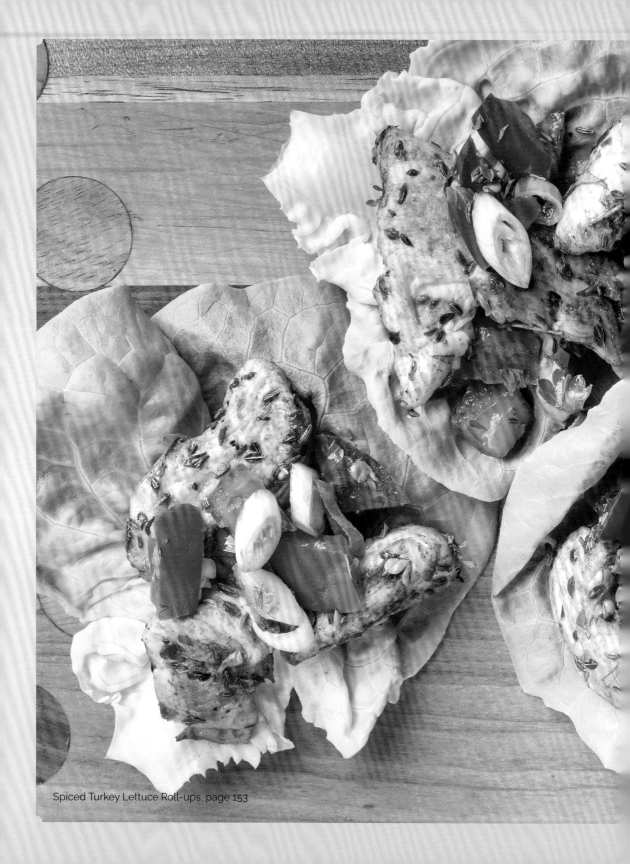

Spiced Turkey Lettuce Roll-ups, page 153

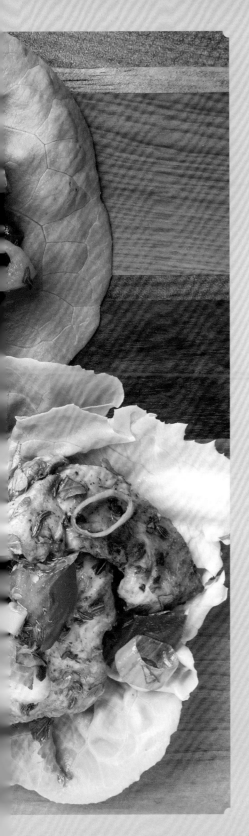

sandwiches, wraps, and handheld meals

These sandwiches, wraps, and handheld meals are nutritious, delicious, and easy to prepare. They are also very satisfying because of the balanced carbohydrates, proteins, and fats, so you won't get sleepy or have a sugar crash in the afternoon. My favorite recipe in this chapter is the power-packed Amazing Avocado Toast. I exercise a lot, and this dish keeps my energy levels up even when I am working out.

amazing avocado toast

Some may think that this is only a trendy food, but I'm convinced it will stand the test of time. It's an easy and delicious lunch and the egg on top makes it a complete meal. You can tailor it to your taste and cook the egg just the way you like it.

Makes 1 serving

1 tbsp | 15 mL ghee

1 large egg

½ avocado

Salt and black pepper

2 cherry tomatoes, quartered

¼ green onion, chopped finely

1 slice rye bread, toasted

Cook the egg however you like it. For sunny-side up, heat the ghee in a nonstick skillet over low heat. Carefully crack the egg into the skillet, cover, and cook until the white is set but the yolk is runny, 2–3 minutes.

Meanwhile, in a medium bowl, mash the avocado with salt to taste. Add the tomatoes and green onion and mix well.

To assemble, spread the avocado mixture on the toast and top with the egg. Season with salt and pepper to taste.

Getting Back to 3 Square Meals

There are no between-meal options on the Metabolic Balance plan because the body needs time to balance insulin levels. That means only 3 meals per day. If you find yourself getting hungry between meals, drink more water or go for a walk. You will be surprised how quickly your hunger disappears. However, it will also help to choose meals that have higher fats, like avocado, cheese, eggs, and meats. After reaching your goal weight, you will be able to eat more food and will find your body completely adjusts to eating 3 meals a day.

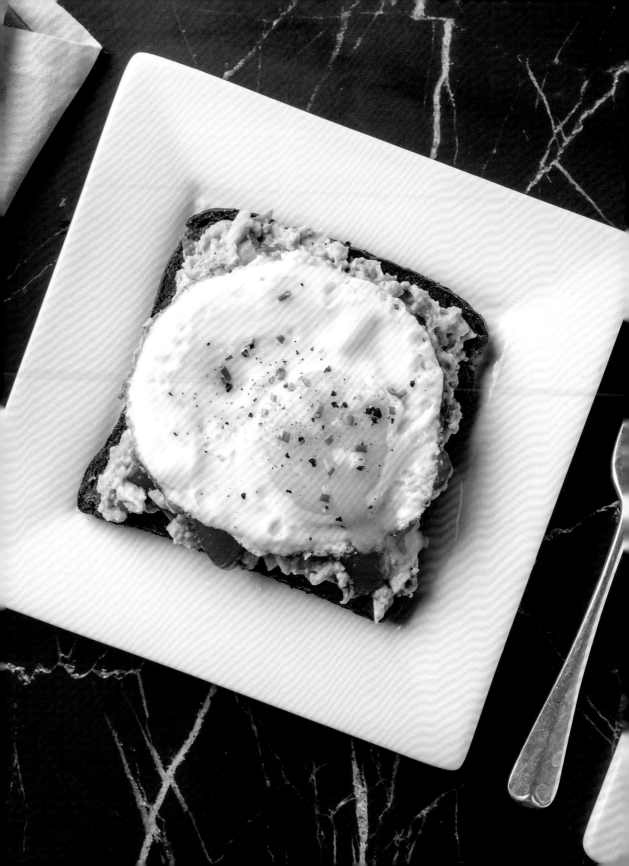

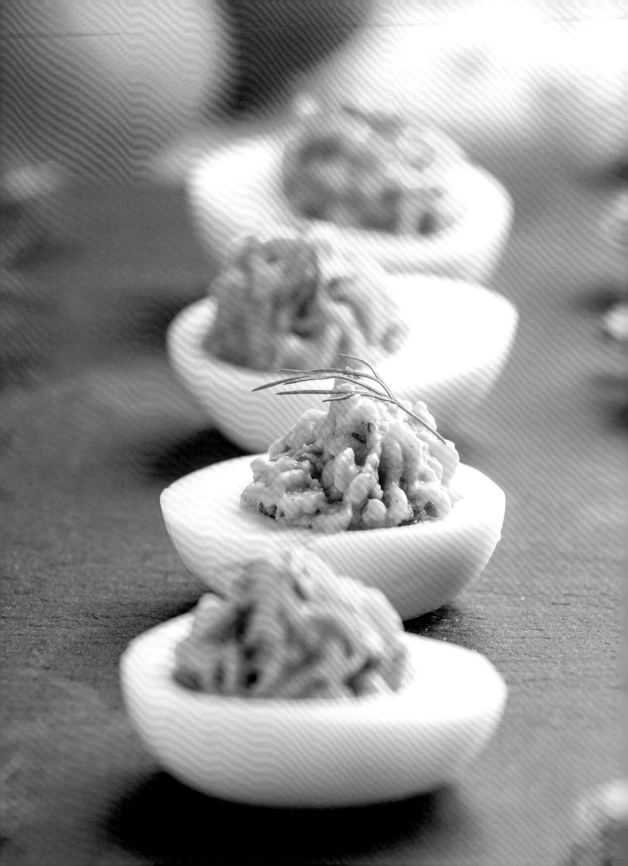

avocado deviled eggs
with greens

Eggs provide one of the highest value sources of protein, and these deviled eggs have a spicy kick with the addition of jalapeño and mustard. To make this a meal, serve over a bed of greens or enjoy with a small side salad with balsamic vinegar and olive oil. In addition, you should eat 1 apple every day on the Metabolic Balance plan, and a sliced apple would go great with this dish at lunch.

Makes 2 servings

4 large eggs

½ avocado

1 tbsp minced fresh cilantro leaves

1½ tbsp thinly sliced green onion

½ tsp minced jalapeño pepper (optional)

1 tsp | 5 mL grainy mustard

1 tsp salt, or to taste

Lemon or lime juice (optional)

Fill a large saucepan with enough water to cover 4 eggs. Bring to a boil, then carefully add the eggs to the saucepan. Reduce the heat to low and simmer for 10 minutes.

Pour out the hot water and run cold water over the eggs to stop them from cooking any further. Allow them to cool.

Peel the eggs and cut each one in half lengthwise. Remove the yolks and put them in a bowl; set aside the whites.

Add the avocado, cilantro, green onion, jalapeño (if using), mustard, and salt to the yolks and mash until smooth. (If you are not eating the deviled eggs right away, add a squirt of lemon or lime juice to prevent the avocado from browning.)

Fill the empty egg white halves with the avocado mixture, using a piping bag or a small spoon.

Serve right away, or cover and refrigerate until ready to serve.

bibb lettuce roll-ups
with chicken

I often eat light meals at lunch and breakfast and then have a hearty dinner with the family, and this refreshing wrap makes for a lovely lunch. The textures of apple and celery combine and complement each other well, as in a Waldorf salad. Enjoy it with rye bread or rye crackers.

Makes 1 serving

5 oz | 140 g boneless, skinless chicken breast

1 tbsp | 15 mL olive oil

½ tsp dried oregano

½ tsp dried thyme

½ medium tart apple, cut into small dice

½ celery rib, cut into small dice

½ avocado, cubed

1 tbsp | 15 mL apple cider vinegar

½ tsp | 2.5 mL yellow or grain mustard

1 tsp finely chopped fresh parsley

3 or 4 Bibb lettuce leaves

2 rye crackers (such as Wasa or Ryvita) or 1 slice rye bread, toasted

Cut the chicken into bite-size pieces.

Heat the olive oil in a small skillet over medium-high heat. Add the chicken, season with the oregano and thyme, and stir-fry until cooked through, about 10 minutes. Transfer to a medium bowl and allow to cool.

Add the apple, celery, avocado, vinegar, mustard, and parsley to the bowl with the chicken and mix well. Spoon the mixture onto the lettuce leaves and roll them up. Serve with rye crackers or toast.

About the Ingredient: Bibb Lettuce

Bibb lettuce is considered by some to be one of the healthiest of the lettuces. It is rich in vitamins K, B, C, and A and an excellent source of calcium, potassium, and magnesium.

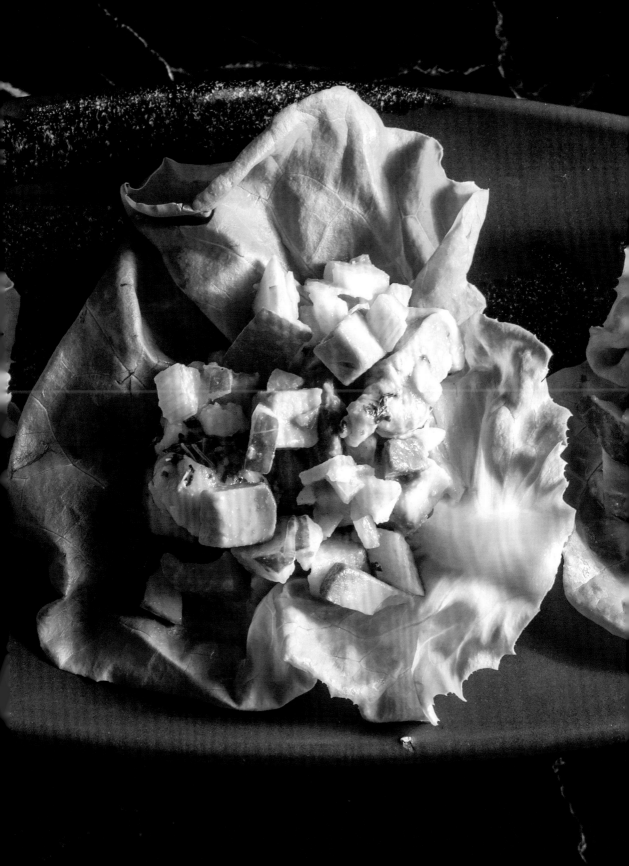

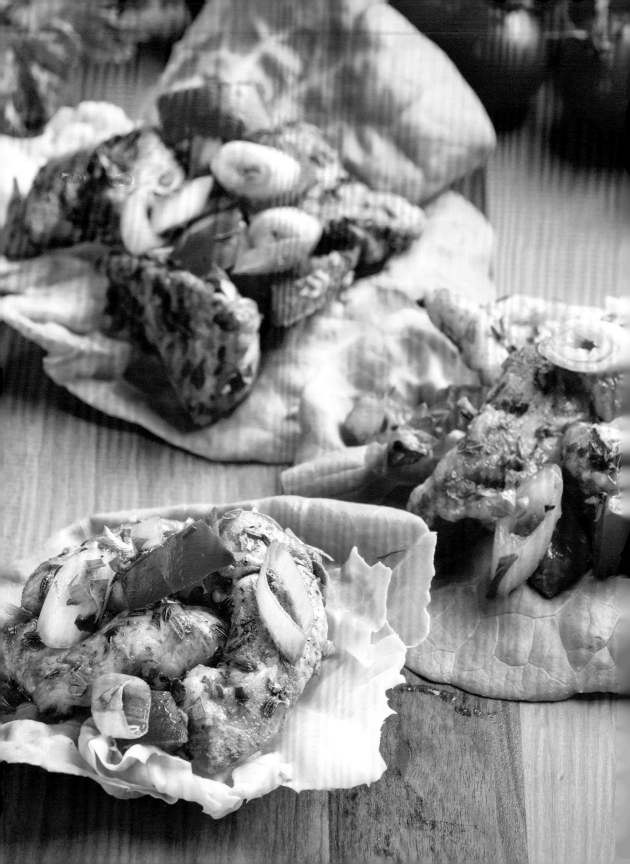

spiced turkey
lettuce roll-ups

My favorite poultry is turkey. Here in North America, it is associated mainly with holidays, but turkey is available at any time of the year. This dish provides a quick lunch that is full of flavor, as well as high in selenium and low in fat.

Makes 1 serving

5 oz | 140 g boneless, skinless turkey breast

2 garlic cloves, finely chopped

⅛ tsp red pepper flakes

⅛ tsp dried thyme

⅛ tsp caraway seeds

⅛ tsp ground allspice

⅛ tsp paprika

1 tbsp | 15 mL coconut oil

6 cherry tomatoes, chopped

2 large Bibb lettuce leaves

½ green onion, thinly sliced

Finely chopped fresh parsley

Salt and black pepper

Slice the turkey into thin strips.

In a small bowl, toss the turkey with the garlic, red pepper flakes, thyme, caraway, allspice, and paprika.

Heat the oil in a small skillet over medium heat. Add the turkey and stir-fry until cooked through, about 6 minutes.

Divide the turkey and chopped tomatoes evenly onto the lettuce leaves. Top with the green onion and parsley and season with salt and pepper to taste. Roll up the lettuce wraps and serve.

The Importance of Hydration

Drinking water throughout the day is vital to keep your metabolic rate high. Within 10 minutes of drinking 2 cups | 475 mL of water, your metabolic rate goes up. In less than one hour, your rate may increase by 30 percent. With an increased metabolic rate, you burn more calories, leading to weight loss.

SANDWICHES, WRAPS, AND HANDHELD MEALS

black-eyed peas
and crackers

This tasty lunch is a great way to get your protein from a nonmeat source without a lot of preparation. Black-eyed peas offer a high source of fiber and protein with a low glycemic load that stabilizes your blood sugar. This is true of other legumes as well, since they contain complex carbohydrates. Black-eyed peas are economical and readily available, and can be prepared in many ways.

Makes 1 serving

1 tbsp | 15 mL olive oil

¼ small onion, chopped

1 cup | 170 g canned black-eyed peas, drained and rinsed

2 tbsp | 30 mL vegetable broth

½ jalapeño pepper, finely chopped

1 tbsp finely chopped red bell pepper

1 small garlic clove, minced

Salt and black pepper

2 rye crackers (such as Wasa or Ryvita) or 1 slice rye bread, toasted

Heat the oil in a small skillet over medium heat. Add the onion and cook until tender, about 2 minutes. Add the black-eyed peas, broth, jalapeño, bell pepper, and garlic. Season with salt and pepper to taste and cook until heated through, about 3 minutes.

Scoop the mixture onto the crackers.

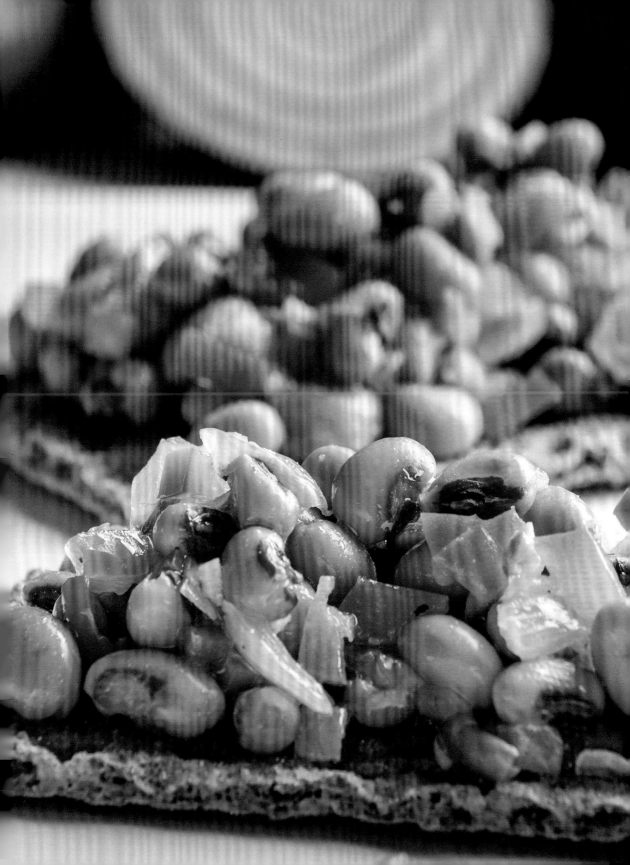

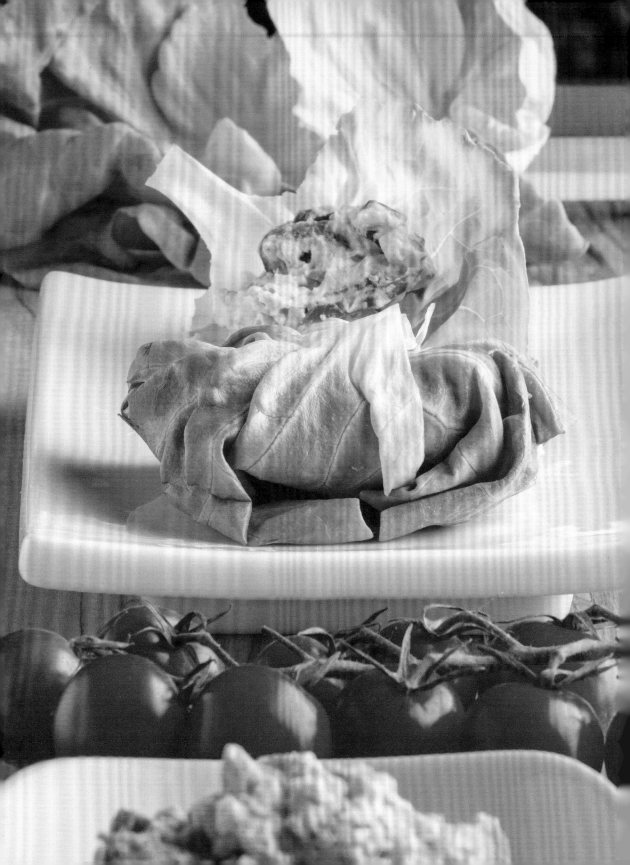

goat cheese and veggie **roll-ups**

The creamy cheese filling for these fresh-tasting rolls needs 1 hour to firm up in the refrigerator after you prepare it. I like to make it in the morning so it's ready to go at lunch. You can also spread it on rye crackers instead of lettuce leaves. Goat cheese is readily available worldwide and is a great source of calcium, which supports the strength and structure of our bones.

Makes 1 serving

½ cup | 80 g goat cheese

½ avocado

1 medium tomato,
seeded and diced

1 green onion,
thinly sliced

2 tbsp diced cucumber

½ tsp dried thyme

Salt and black pepper

2–4 large
Bibb lettuce leaves

In a medium bowl, mash together the goat cheese, avocado, tomato, and green onion. Add the cucumber and season with the thyme and salt and pepper to taste.

Cover and refrigerate for at least 1 hour to firm up.

When you're ready to eat, scoop a large spoonful onto each lettuce leaf and roll them up.

You Can Do It

Making a change in the way you eat can take time, but it is really quite simple with Metabolic Balance. Although there is no magic pill, there is a magic process. Simply adding the 8 Rules of Metabolic Balance to your daily regime can make the transition easy and help you lose weight fast. See pages 34, 39, 60, 65, 131, and 206 for the 8 Rules of Metabolic Balance!

SANDWICHES, WRAPS,
AND HANDHELD MEALS

open-faced
roast beef sandwich

When you're longing to go to New York City and pop into one of their famous delis, this lunch can help satisfy that craving. Deli meats often contain chemical preservatives, heavy oils, and sugar, so I suggest using leftovers from last night's roast for this recipe. Mustard adds a burst of flavor and is a great source of heart-healthy omega-3 fatty acids, along with several antioxidants and anti-inflammatory benefits.

Makes 1 serving

2 rye crackers
(such as Ryvita or Wasa)

2 tsp | 10 mL
coarse-ground mustard

4 oz | 120 g sliced
roast beef

½ tomato, sliced

2 thin slices red onion

Handful arugula leaves

Salt and black pepper

Place the crackers on a plate. Spread the mustard on the crackers. Layer with the roast beef, tomato, onion, and arugula. Season with salt and pepper to taste.

Broiling option: Place crackers on a small rimmed baking sheet and top with the other ingredients, as shown opposite. Preheat the broiler with a rack in the top third of the oven.

Broil on low heat for 2–3 minutes, until warmed.

An Apple a Day . . .

This is a great meal to enjoy with 1 sliced tart apple. Apples are delicious served alongside a variety of recipes, and it's important to eat 1 whole tart apple per day with a meal.

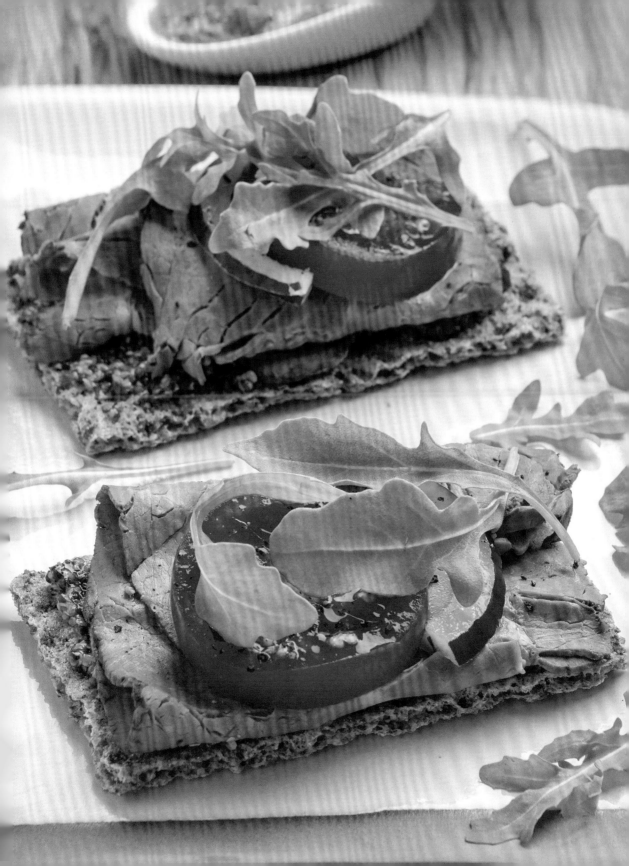

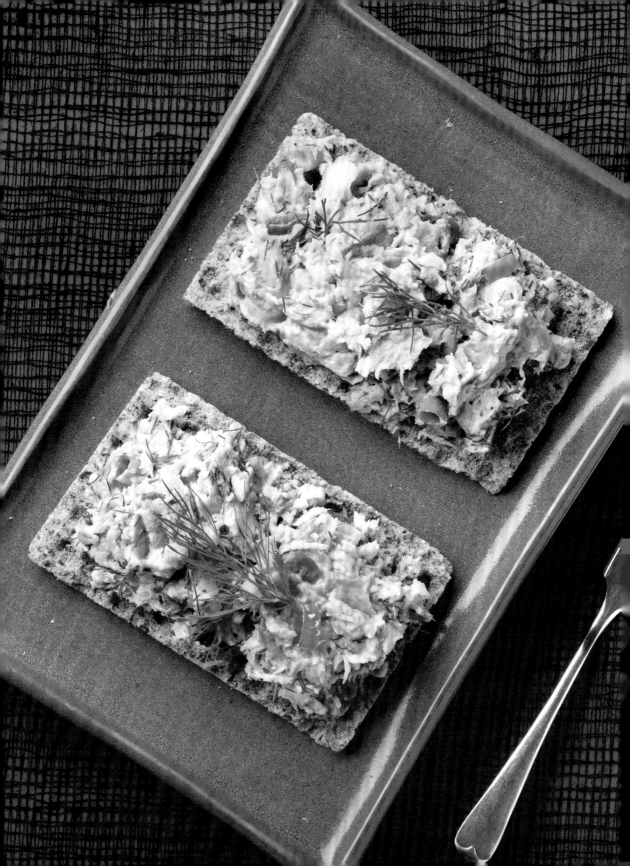

fish spread
and rye crackers

The American Heart Association recommends eating fish because they are a concentrated source of omega-3 fatty acids, which are a great energy source and keep the heart and immune system working well. When I'm in a hurry at lunchtime, I love this flavorful salmon dish because it takes almost no time to prepare.

Makes 1 serving

½ avocado

1 (5-oz | 140 g) can salmon, drained

2 tbsp finely chopped green onion

2 tbsp chopped fresh dill

Salt and black pepper

2 rye crackers (such as Ryvita or Wasa) or 1 slice rye bread, toasted

Fresh dill leaves, for garnish (optional)

In a medium bowl, mash the avocado. Add the salmon, flaking it apart. Add the green onion and dill and mix until creamy. Season with salt and pepper to taste. Scoop onto the rye crackers. Garnish with fresh dill, if desired.

salmon and avocado
open-faced sandwich

This wonderful open-faced sandwich is extremely satisfying. The protein in the salmon and the fat in the avocado maintain your blood sugar balance and keep insulin at a healthy level.

Makes 1 serving

4½ oz | 130 g
salmon fillet

½ avocado

¼ red onion,
finely chopped

½ celery rib,
finely chopped

1 tbsp finely chopped
fresh dill, plus more
for garnish

Salt and black pepper

1 slice rye bread,
toasted if desired,
or 2 rye crackers
(such as Wasa or Ryvita)

In a small skillet, sear the salmon over medium-high heat until just cooked through, 2–3 minutes on each side. Transfer the salmon to a plate and allow to cool.

In a small bowl, mash the avocado, then add the onion, celery, and dill and mix well. Add the salmon to the avocado mixture, breaking it apart with a fork into bite-size pieces.

Season with salt and pepper to taste and spread on the rye bread.

Add fresh dill as garnish, if desired.

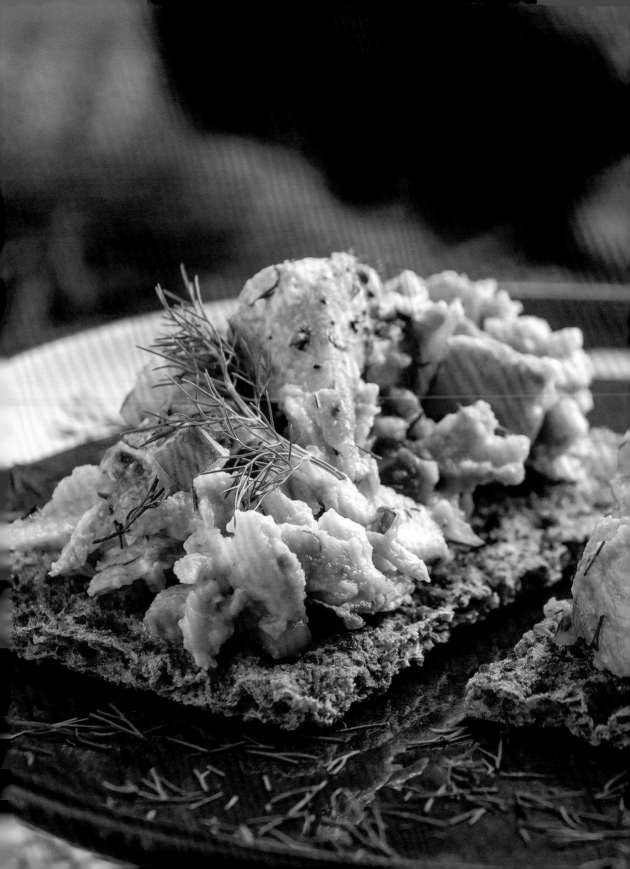

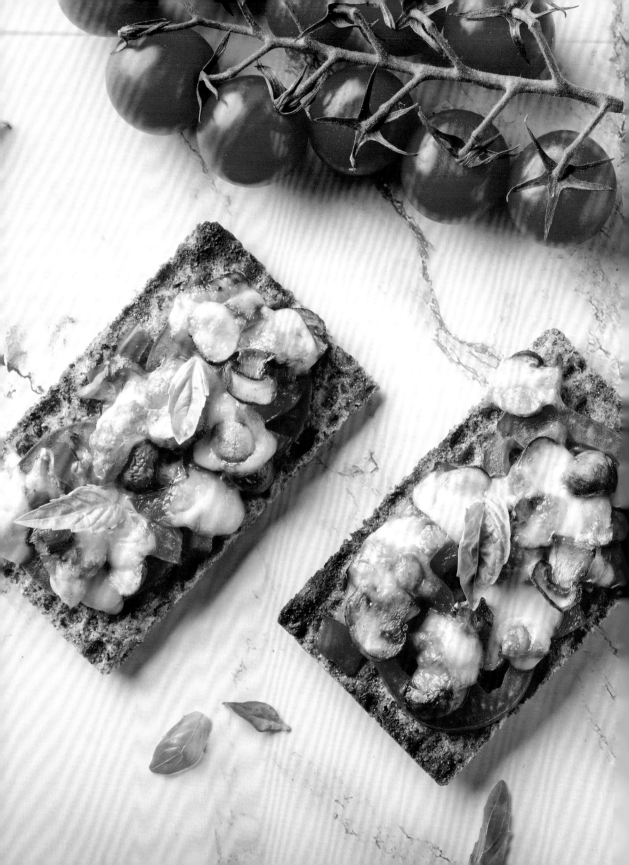

cheese and veggie **pizza**

Yes, you can eat pizza on the Metabolic Balance program—as long as it is this yummy pizza with a rye-cracker base! You won't feel bloated or sluggish after eating this, and the toppings are so flavorful that you'll never miss the pepperoni.

Makes 1 serving

1 tsp | 5 mL
olive oil

1 garlic clove, minced

2 button mushrooms,
cut into small dice

1 Roma tomato,
thinly sliced

½ medium onion,
cut into small dice

¼ red bell pepper,
cut into small dice

Pinch dried oregano

Pinch dried or chopped
fresh basil

2 rye crackers (such as
Wasa or Ryvita) or 1 slice
rye bread, toasted

½ cup | 80 g mozzarella
balls (bocconcini) or
crumbled goat cheese

Preheat the broiler with a rack in the top third of the oven.

Heat the oil in a small skillet over medium-high heat. Add the garlic and sauté until golden, about 1 minute. Add the mushrooms, tomato, onion, and bell pepper and cook for 2 minutes, then flip the vegetables, sprinkle with the herbs, and cook until softened, about 2 minutes more.

Place the rye crackers on a small rimmed baking sheet. Put one-quarter of the cheese on each cracker. Top with the vegetable mixture. Scatter the remaining cheese over each.

Broil until the cheese melts, 2–3 minutes. Enjoy warm.

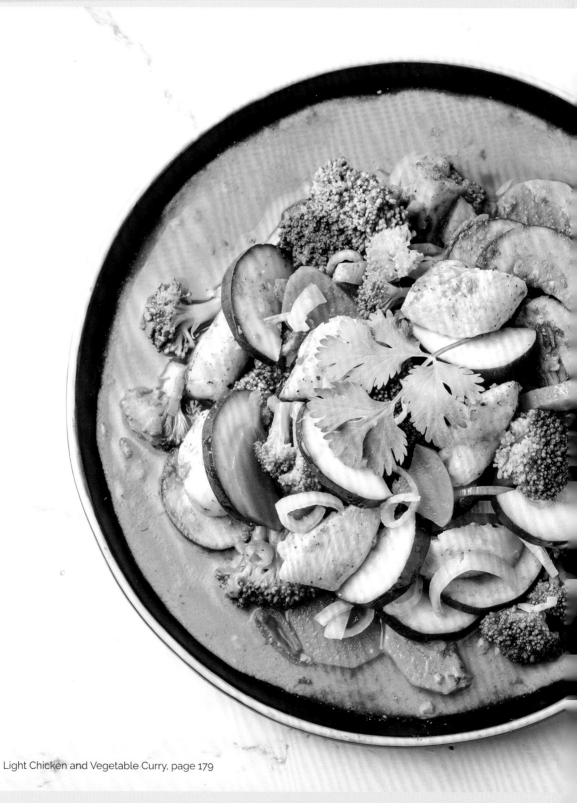

Light Chicken and Vegetable Curry, page 179

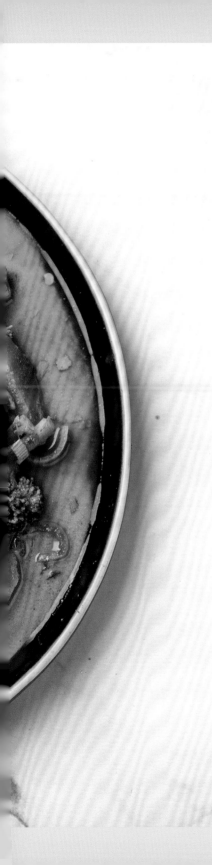

main dishes

At my house, dinner is a time for people to come together and enjoy food and conversation. When you're eating the Metabolic Balance way, dinner is especially important, because when you're finished, you'll fast until breakfast. We still need energy for those 8 to 12 hours while winding down for the night and sleeping, and having a dinner with the right balance of protein, fats, and carbs ensures we will wake up feeling energized, happy, and ready for the day. While many of the recipes in the earlier chapters can make for a delicious dinner, the poultry, meat, and seafood dishes in this chapter are specially created for a satisfying evening meal that will hold you over nicely until morning. The recipes in this chapter that serve 1 person can easily be doubled or quadrupled to feed a couple or a hungry family. Some of my favorites are the Chicken Breast with Spicy Basil Sauce and Zucchini, the Creamy Eggplant and Lamb Stew, and the Crispy Blackened Salmon. Take time to enjoy and savor every mouthful.

chicken breast with spicy basil sauce and zucchini

This spicy chicken with pungent basil sauce awakens your senses with a burst of flavor and will become an instant favorite. If you'd prefer it mild, the dish can be made without the Thai chile with no loss of flavor. The sauce and zucchini also make a wonderful accompaniment for fish fillets (try them with my Crispy Blackened Salmon, page 194).

Makes 1 serving

Chicken Breast

4 oz | 115 g boneless, skinless chicken breast

1 tsp | 5 mL lemon juice

1 tbsp | 15 mL olive oil

Sauce and Zucchini

2 tbsp chopped fresh basil, divided, plus whole leaves for garnish (optional)

1 Thai chile, finely chopped, divided

1 tbsp finely chopped red bell pepper, divided

1 tbsp fresh parsley leaves

1 tsp | 5 mL lemon juice

2 tbsp | 10 mL olive oil

Salt and black pepper

½ medium zucchini, spiralized

1–2 cauliflower florets, crumbled

In a small dish, marinate the chicken breast with 1 tsp | 5 ml lemon juice and 1 tbsp | 15 mL oil for 1 hour.

Preheat the broiler and position an oven rack in the top third of your oven. Place the chicken on a baking sheet. Broil for 6 minutes per side until lightly browned and cooked through. Remove and slice chicken into strips.

In a small food processor, combine half of the basil, half of the chile, half of the bell pepper, the parsley, lemon juice, and oil, and season to taste with salt and pepper. Pulse until everything is well combined and chopped very small. Place in a small saucepan and heat on low for 5–6 minutes.

In a nonstick, medium frying pan over high heat, stir-fry the zucchini and cauliflower with the remaining basil, chile, and bell pepper for 5 minutes until softened.

Place the sliced chicken on a dinner plate and arrange the zucchini mixture alongside. Drizzle the warmed basil sauce over the chicken and zucchini and garnish with basil, if desired.

TIP: Spiralizers are inexpensive and so worth it! You can have perfect zucchini noodles every time. Thicker noodles are best because they hold their shape and don't become mushy. Spiralize the zucchini, salt it lightly, and let it rest for at least 20 minutes. That will allow a lot of the water to be released. Then pat the noodles dry with paper towels, toss them into a skillet, and cook until tender, stirring often.

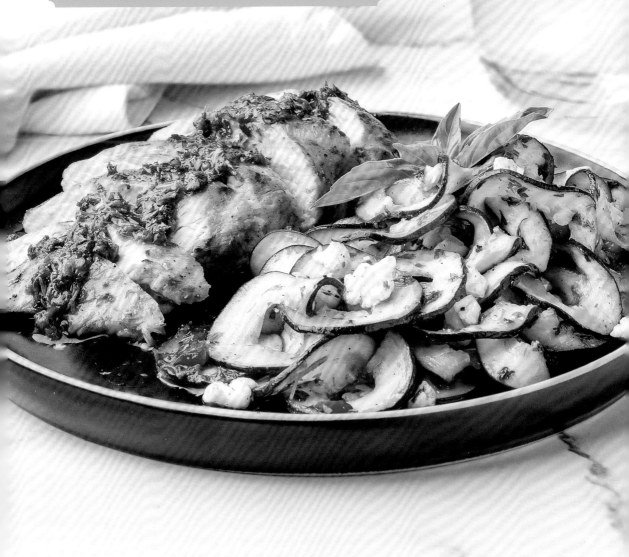

ginger chicken stir-fry

When you take your first bite of this flavorful chicken dish, your taste buds will dance with the pungent, aromatic taste of the ginger. Fresh ginger should be firm, with a shiny and smooth skin. Avoid ginger that is wrinkled, soft, or cracked as it has lost most of its flavor and pungency.

Makes 1 serving

5 oz | 140 g boneless, skinless chicken breast

1 tbsp | 15 mL olive oil

½ onion, cut into small dice

1 small red chile pepper, seeded and finely chopped

1 garlic clove, minced

2 button mushrooms, sliced

1 (1-in | 2.5-cm) piece fresh ginger, cut into fine strips

1 tomato, diced

1 tbsp | 15 mL vegetable broth or water

Black pepper

1 tbsp chopped fresh cilantro leaves

1 tsp sesame seeds, for garnish

Cut the chicken breast into bite-size pieces.

In a large skillet or wok, heat the oil over medium-high heat. Add the onion, chile, and garlic and sauté until the onion is almost translucent, about 2 minutes. Add the chicken and stir-fry until evenly browned, 3–5 minutes. Add the mushrooms and ginger and continue stir-frying until the mushrooms are softened and the chicken is cooked through, another 3–5 minutes. Add the tomato and broth and season with pepper to taste. Give the dish a final toss to heat through.

Sprinkle with the cilantro and garnish with the sesame seeds.

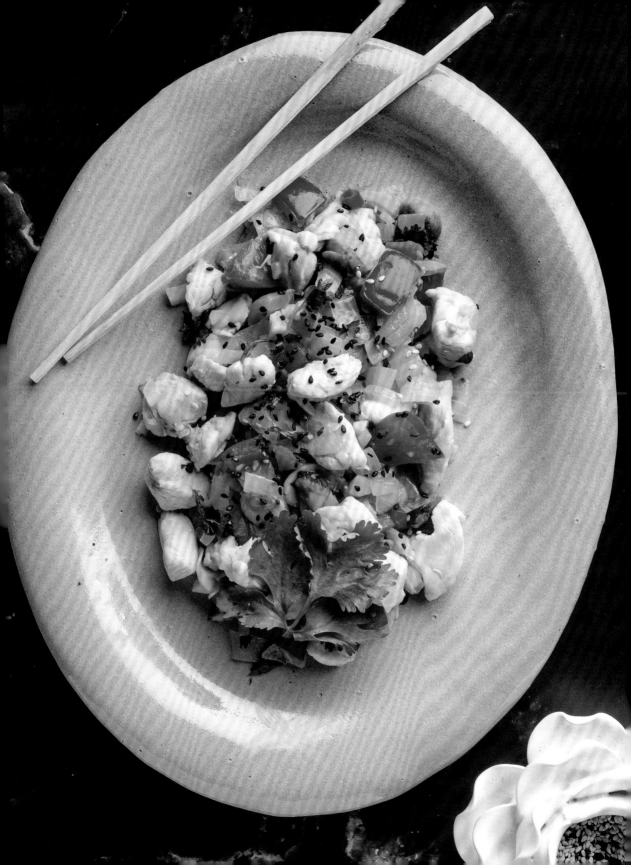

dijon chicken with
pesto asparagus pasta

treat meal

This is a special dish. My granddaughters, Lauren and Rachel, come for dinner every Sunday and when I tell them I'm making this dish, they always ask me to make extra so they can take it home for their lunch the next day. I love pesto, as I like to eat my greens and other vegetables raw as much as possible. It is only gently heated to preserve the nutrients in the basil leaves. The recipe makes about 3 cups of pesto. You will use 1 cup in this recipe and can freeze the remainder to enjoy later.

Makes 4 servings

Chicken

4 (6-oz | 170-g) bone-in, skin-on chicken breasts

½ cup | 120 mL Dijon mustard

Juice of 1 lemon

Pesto Pasta

1 bunch asparagus, ends trimmed

Place the chicken breasts in a large bowl. Add the mustard and lemon juice and toss until the chicken breasts are fully coated in the mixture. Cover and refrigerate for at least 1 hour, or overnight.

Preheat the oven to 350°F | 175°C.

Transfer the chicken to a small baking dish and bake for 45 minutes, or until the chicken skin is looks brown and crispy. Once cooled, cut into bite-size pieces and set aside.

Meanwhile, fill a large pot with water and bring to a boil. Add the asparagus and boil for 2 minutes, or until crisp-tender. Using tongs, transfer the asparagus to a cutting board and allow to cool slightly; reserve the pot of hot water. When cool enough to handle, cut the asparagus into bite-size pieces and set aside.

Ingredients and directions continued on next page ▶

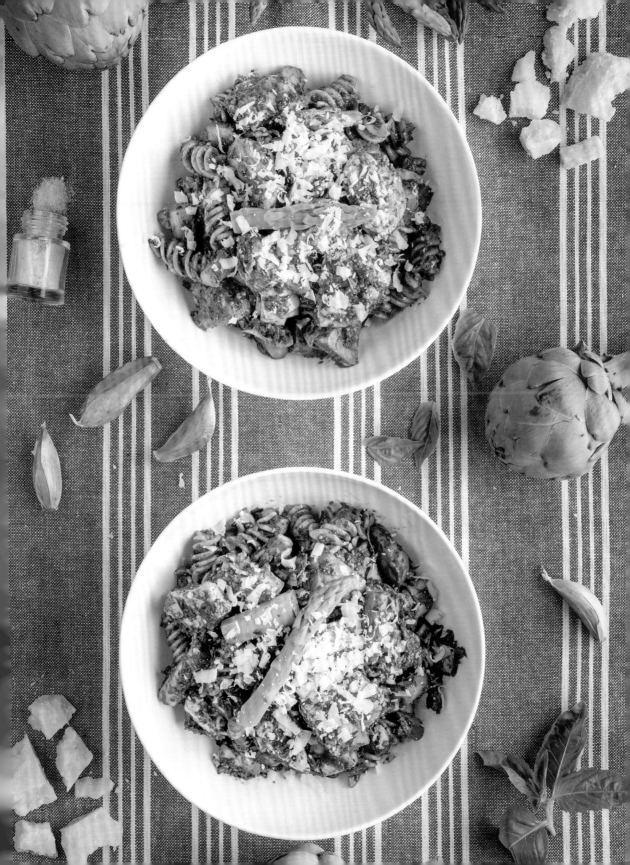

4 tbsp | 57 g butter

6 garlic cloves, peeled

1 cup | 100 g raw
walnut halves

¾ cup | 180 mL olive oil

1¼ cups | 100 g coarsely
grated Parmesan cheese

½ tsp salt

½ tsp black pepper

8 bunches basil, leaves
removed from stems

2–4 tbsp | 30–60 mL
water, as needed

1 cup | 170 g marinated
artichoke hearts, drained
and roughly chopped

1 pound | 454 g
brown rice fusilli pasta

Melt the butter in a medium saucepan over low heat. Set aside to cool slightly, then transfer the melted butter to a food processor; do not wipe out the saucepan. Add the garlic, walnuts, oil, Parmesan, salt, pepper, and half the basil leaves. Whizz the ingredients for about 30 seconds, then scrape down the sides, add the rest of the basil, and whizz again until smooth, about 30 seconds more. Add a few tablespoons of water if it's too thick.

Transfer the pesto to the reserved saucepan. Add the chicken, artichoke hearts, and asparagus and toss to coat well. Cook over low heat for 10 minutes, stirring often so it does not stick or burn, until heated through.

Return the pot of water to a boil. Cook the pasta according to the package directions. Drain the pasta, then return it to the pot.

Add the chicken, asparagus, artichoke, and pesto mixture to the pasta. Cook over medium heat, stirring often, for 30 seconds to 1 minute to warm the entire mixture.

About the Ingredient: Basil

Basil is a tender herb that is used in cuisines around the world. A source of healthy volatile oil and phytonutrients, it is used to aid digestion as well as to flavor food, and it is both naturally antibacterial and anti-inflammatory. It is considered by some to be the king of herbs, and is a concentrated source of iron, calcium, fiber, vitamins A and C, and potassium.

mouthwatering
curry chicken

Though coconut milk is not on personalized Metabolic Balance plans, I had to include this nourishing curry bowl in the cookbook. It may look complicated, but this dish takes just moments to make. The combination of spices makes the coconut milk base delicious. This curry tastes amazing over warm quinoa or any rice of your choice.

Makes 4 servings

3 (4-oz | 115-g) boneless, skinless chicken breasts

2 tbsp | 30 mL coconut oil or olive oil

2 garlic cloves, minced

1 (1-in | 2.5-cm) piece ginger, grated

2 tbsp ground coriander

1 tsp ground cumin

1 tsp salt

½ tsp ground turmeric

½ tsp ground cinnamon

½ tsp cayenne pepper

¼ tsp ground cardamom

¼ tsp ground cloves

2 medium yellow onions, diced

1½ cups | 355 mL coconut milk

½ green onion, chopped

1 tbsp unsweetened shredded or flaked coconut, for garnish

Chop the chicken breasts into bite-size pieces and set aside.

Heat the oil in a wok or large skillet over medium heat. Add the garlic and ginger and stir-fry until fragrant, about 1 minute. Add the coriander, cumin, salt, turmeric, cinnamon, cayenne, cardamom, and cloves and stir constantly for 1 minute to distribute evenly in the oil, being careful not to let the spices burn.

Stir in the onions and toss to coat in the spiced oil. Cook until tender, 2–3 minutes. Add the chicken and coconut milk and bring to a boil. Reduce the heat and simmer for 15 minutes, or until the chicken is cooked through. Add the green onion and garnish with the coconut.

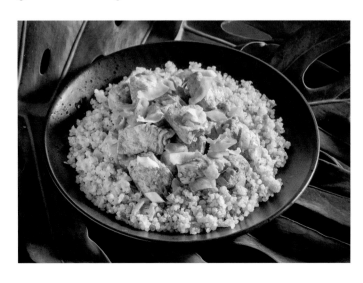

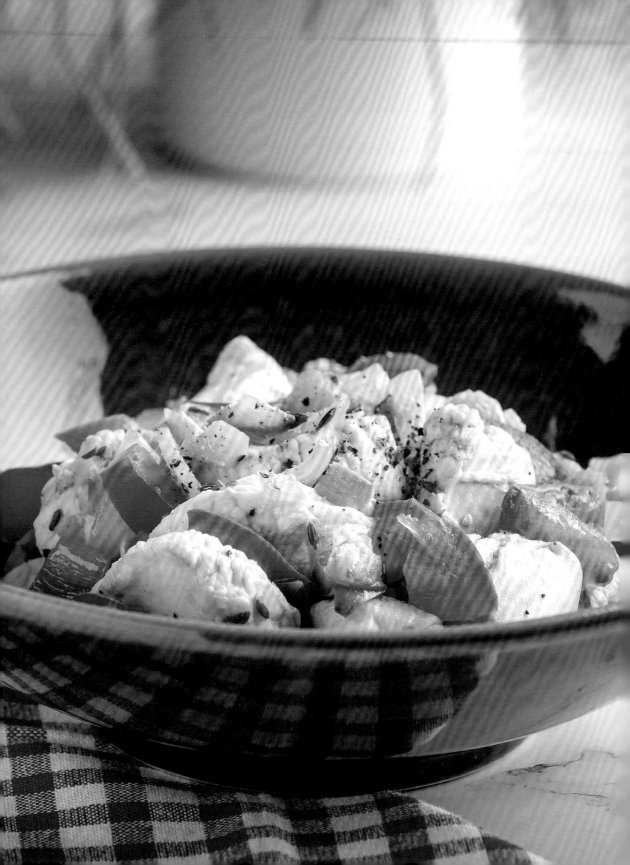

green onion and tomato
chicken

I love this dish! It is bright, fresh, and chock-full of flavor—plus, it looks elegant but is easy and quick to prepare. Chicken is a staple for many people worldwide and an excellent protein source. Enjoy this dish with a small side salad, 2 rye crackers, and 1 cup fresh mango cubes.

Makes 1 serving

4½ oz | 130 g boneless, skinless chicken breast

¼ tsp cumin seeds

½ onion, chopped

1 (1-in | 2.5-cm) piece fresh ginger, grated

1 small garlic clove, minced

1 green chile pepper, finely chopped

1 Roma tomato, diced

1 green onion, sliced

¼ tsp chili powder

Salt and black pepper

½ cup | 120 mL water

Cut the chicken breast into bite-size pieces. Set aside.

Heat a medium skillet over low heat. Add the cumin and toast until golden and fragrant, about 2 minutes. Add the onion and stir-fry until translucent, about 2 minutes. Add the ginger, garlic, and chile and stir-fry for 30 seconds.

Add the chicken, increase the heat to medium, and stir-fry until the meat is seared on the outside, 5–7 minutes. Add the tomato, green onion, and chili powder. Season with salt and pepper to taste.

Add the water, reduce the heat to low, and simmer for 15 minutes, or until the chicken is cooked through.

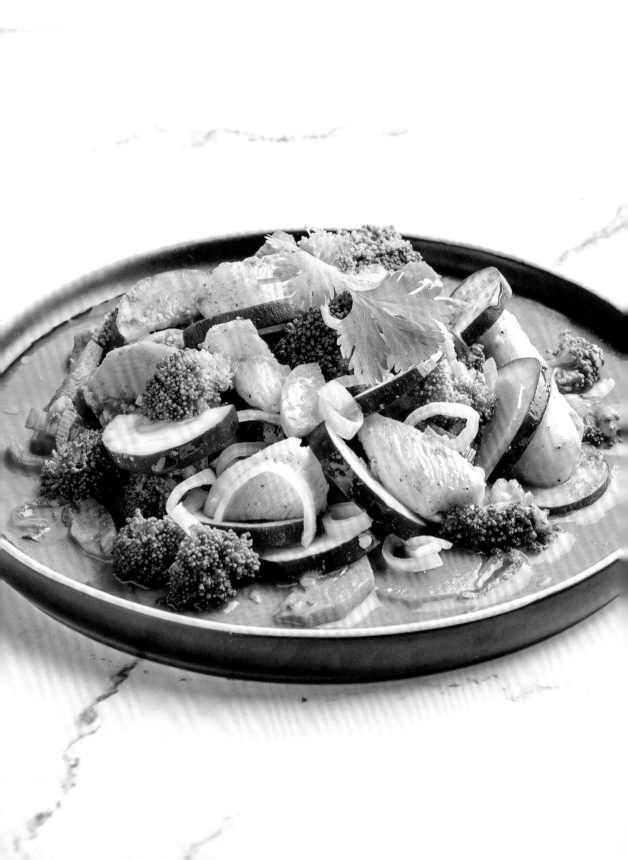

light chicken and vegetable **curry**

This light and delectable curry is loaded with minerals and other nutrients. Turmeric, the main spice in most curry dishes, has anti-inflammatory properties. This recipe is a favorite of my family and is full of fresh vegetables and bursting with flavor. You can also use any firm white fish in this recipe instead of chicken.

Makes 1 serving

5 oz | 140 g boneless, skinless chicken breast

⅔ cup | 160 mL water, plus more as needed

1 (1-in | 2.5-cm) piece fresh ginger, minced

1 tsp ground turmeric

1 tsp ground cumin

1 tsp paprika

1 tsp ground mustard

⅛ tsp red pepper flakes

½ tsp salt

⅓ cup | 25 g small broccoli florets

⅓ cup | 30 g sliced carrot

⅓ cup | 30 g sliced leek

¼ cup | 30 g sliced zucchini

Cut the chicken breast into bite-size pieces. Set aside.

Heat the water in a medium saucepan over low heat. Add the ginger, turmeric, cumin, paprika, mustard, red pepper flakes, and salt and cook, stirring constantly, for 1 minute. Add the broccoli, carrot, leek, and zucchini and stir. Increase the heat to medium, cover, and cook for about 5 minutes, or until the broccoli is al dente.

Add the chicken. If needed, add up to ½ cup | 120 mL more water (enough to keep the ingredients moist and create a small amount of pan sauce). Cook with the lid slightly ajar until the chicken is tender and cooked through, 5–10 minutes.

spicy **coriander chicken**

india

This hearty chicken dish, provided by Metabolic Balance coaches in India, explodes with exciting favor. Cilantro, also known as coriander in some countries, is full of nutrients including potassium, which is an electrolyte that provides energy. Combined with all the other spices, the fresh herb mellows the flavor and freshens and brightens the chicken. It makes everyday chicken special. Serve hot with steamed cauliflower or the vegetable of your choice.

Makes 2 servings

2 (4-oz | 115-g) boneless, skinless chicken breasts

½ bunch cilantro, roughly chopped

1 small onion, roughly chopped

2–3 garlic cloves, roughly chopped

1 (1-in | 2.5-cm) piece ginger, grated

1 tsp ground coriander

1 tbsp dried fenugreek leaves (known as kasoori methi in India)

1 tsp chili powder

1 tsp garam masala

Salt

1 tbsp | 15 mL water

1 green onion, thinly sliced on the diagonal

Cut the chicken breasts into bite-size pieces.

In a small food processor or mortar and pestle, make a paste with the fresh cilantro, onion, garlic, ginger, and ground coriander. Transfer the mixture to a medium bowl and mix in the dried fenugreek leaves, chili powder, garam masala, and salt to taste. Add the chicken and toss to thoroughly coat the pieces with the mixture. Cover and refrigerate for at least 1 hour or overnight.

Heat the water in a medium skillet over medium heat. Add the chicken, cover, and cook for 20–25 minutes, until the chicken is almost cooked through. It should be firm but not tough.

Top with the green onion and toss till fully cooked, about 3 more minutes.

TIP: You may also add 3 strips of ripe mango to this recipe, if you like. Marinate the mango along with the chicken, then proceed with the recipe as written.

Special acknowledgment to Seema Malik in India for this recipe.

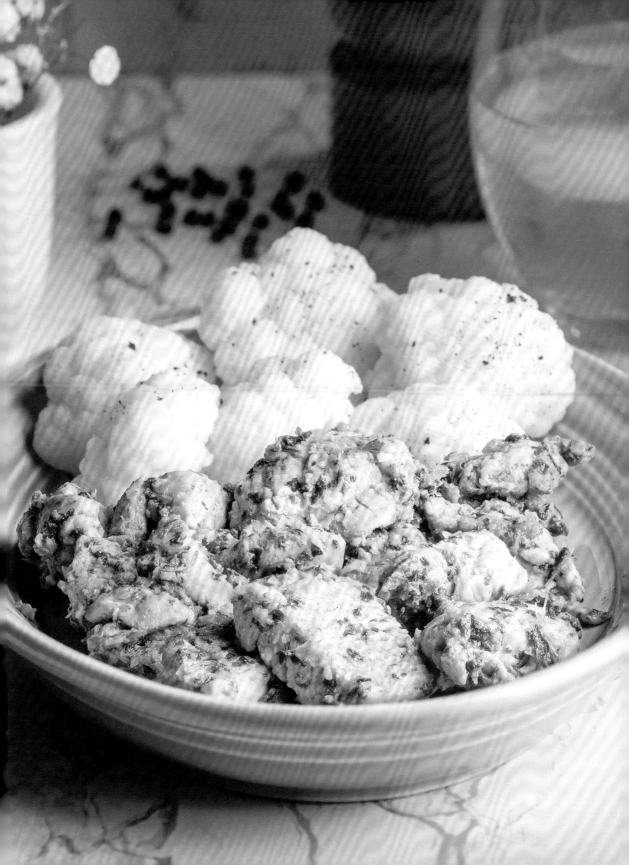

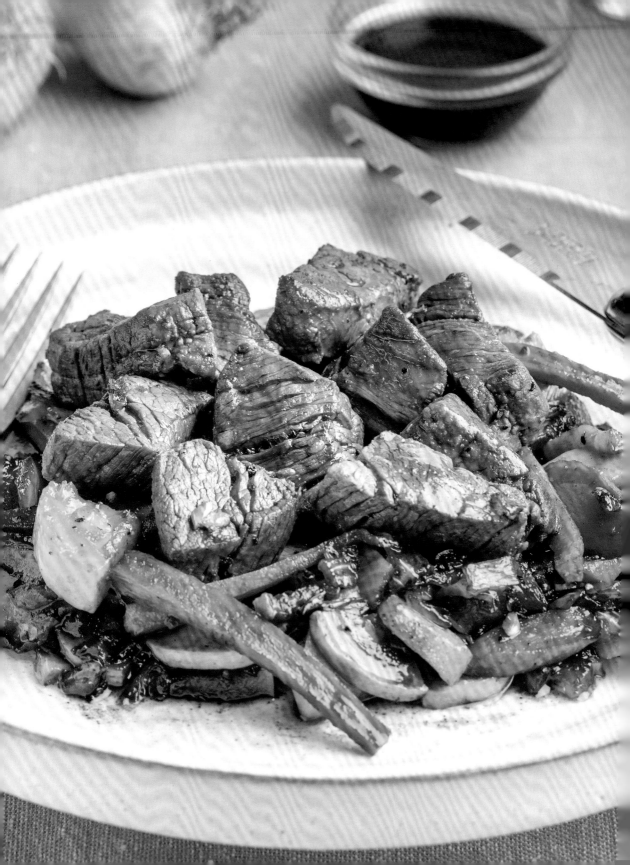

warm **balsamic beef**

This tangy beef dish is one of my favorites—it's mouthwatering and very quick and easy to prepare. The balsamic vinegar provides a hint of sweetness that is totally satisfying to the palate. I love to serve this dish with a bed of salad greens, or you can have it with rye bread or crackers.

Makes 1 serving

5 oz | 140 g beef fillet
or tenderloin

1 tbsp | 15 mL coconut oil

1 tbsp | 15 mL
balsamic vinegar

1 small onion, diced

1 garlic clove, minced

½ yellow zucchini, sliced
into thin half-moons

½ carrot, sliced
into matchsticks

Salt and black pepper

Slice the beef into bite-size pieces.

Heat the oil in a large skillet over medium heat. Stir in the vinegar, onion, and garlic. Add the beef and stir-fry for 3–5 minutes to sear the meat.

Add the zucchini and carrot and stir-fry until the carrot has softened and the beef is tender, 2–3 minutes. Season with salt and pepper to taste.

beef and brussels sprout
stir-fry

Beef and brussels sprouts is a hearty and healthy dish that will definitely satisfy your hunger. It's full of protein, fiber, and phytonutrients. There's a lot of buzz about liver detoxing, and brussels sprouts contain large concentrations of health-promoting sulfur compounds, such as glucosinolates and isothiocyanates, which increase the liver's ability to produce enzymes that neutralize potentially toxic substances. This is a liver-healthy meal!

Makes 1 serving

5 oz | 140 g beef tenderloin

6 medium brussels sprouts

1 tbsp | 15 mL coconut oil

1 garlic clove, minced

¼ tsp dried oregano

¼ tsp cayenne pepper

Salt and black pepper

Chopped fresh cilantro leaves, for garnish

Slice the beef into bite-size pieces. Cut an x on the bottom of each brussels sprout with a paring knife.

Fill a small pot two-thirds full of water. Add the sprouts and cover. Bring to a boil and cook for about 15 minutes, or until a knife can be inserted easily. Drain and let cool.

Heat the oil in a medium skillet over medium heat. Add the beef, garlic, oregano, and cayenne and stir-fry to brown the meat for 4–6 minutes.

Cut the cooled sprouts in quarters and add to the skillet. Continue cooking until the meat is cooked through, 2–3 minutes.

Season with salt and pepper to taste and garnish with cilantro.

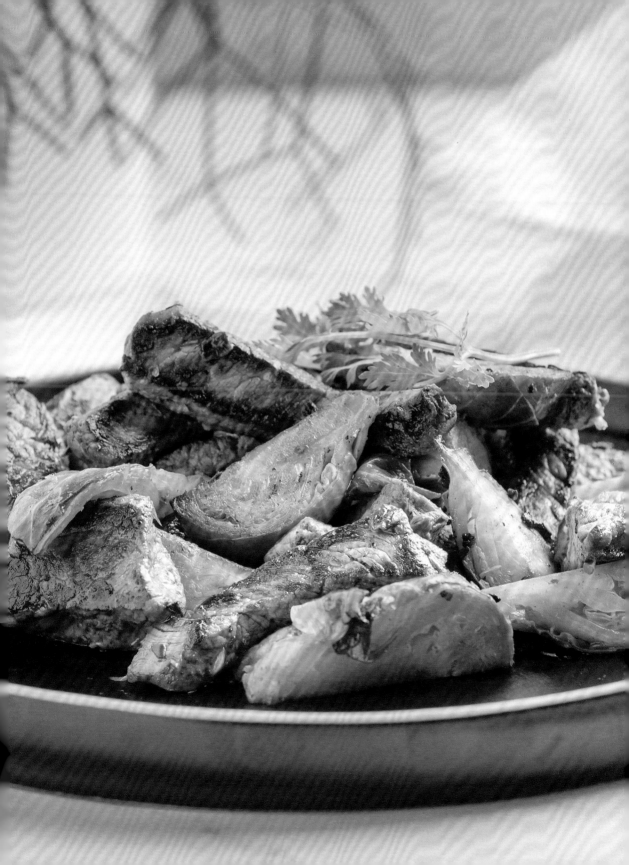

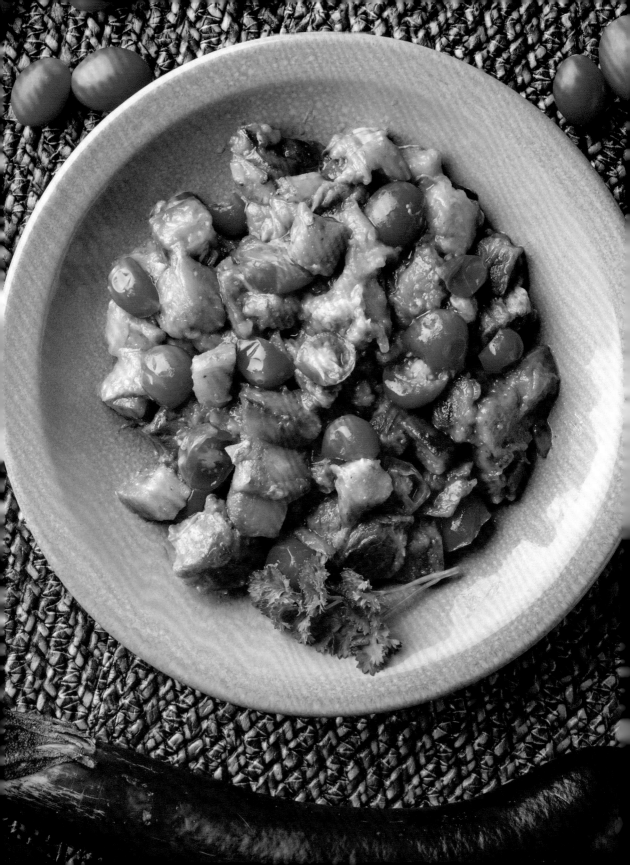

creamy eggplant and lamb stew

iran

It's comforting to have the pleasant aromas of cooking foods wafting through your home. It gives a sense of anticipation of good things to come. This dish from Metabolic Balance coaches in Iran doesn't disappoint. Lamb is my favorite red meat, and it combines so well with creamy eggplant. Lamb is known as one of the finest-tasting meats and it becomes more flavorful when properly prepared.

Makes 1 serving

5 oz | 140 g boneless lamb

½ small white onion, diced

⅛ tsp ground turmeric

Salt and black pepper

1 cup | 240 mL water

1 tsp | 5 mL olive oil

½ small eggplant, peeled and halved lengthwise

5 cherry tomatoes, halved, or ½ tomato, diced

Cut the lamb into bite-size pieces.

In a medium pot, combine the lamb, onion, turmeric, and salt and pepper to taste. Stir-fry over medium-high heat for about 3 minutes, or until the lamb is seared on the outside. Add the water, reduce the heat to low, cover, and simmer for 10 minutes.

Meanwhile, in a nonstick skillet, heat the oil over medium heat. Add the eggplant and stir-fry for about 5 minutes, turning to sear on all sides, until golden brown. Transfer the eggplant to a cutting board and cut into bite-size pieces.

Add the eggplant and tomatoes to the pot with the lamb. Cover and continue to cook over low heat for 30 minutes, or until the lamb is tender. Toward the end of the cooking time, remove the lid if too much liquid remains. Season with salt and pepper to taste.

The Truth About Cholesterol

Almost every cell in the body makes cholesterol, and the liver makes even more to help with the supply and demand. We need cholesterol to build cell membranes, create sex hormones, and make vitamin D from sunlight. Cholesterol is not the problem. Inflammation is! The Metabolic Balance program is designed to fight inflammation every step of the way.

Special acknowledgment to Couros Kamal in Iran for this recipe.

MAIN DISHES

chile pork stir-fry

This stir-fry reminds us why we love this cooking process. When you come home and want to throw something together, this is a perfect fuss-free meal. Plus, the chile pepper not only gives this dish heat but also delivers many health benefits. They are anti-inflammatory, provide pain relief properties, and may help burn excess fat. (And as many of us know from experience, their spice can also help clear congestion!)

Makes 1 serving

5 oz | 140 g pork tenderloin

1 chile pepper, minced

½ tsp ground cumin

1 small garlic clove, minced

Leaves from
1 cilantro sprig

¼ tsp salt

½ tsp | 2.5 mL coconut oil

½ cup | 50 g
cauliflower florets

½ cup | 60 g
sliced zucchini

¼ cup | 60 g sliced
bell pepper

Cut the pork into bite-size pieces and place in a medium bowl. Add the chile, cumin, garlic, cilantro, and salt and toss to coat the pork on all sides with the spices. Cover and refrigerate for at least 45 minutes, or overnight.

Heat the oil in a medium skillet over medium heat. Add the pork and cook until tender and lightly browned, 5–8 minutes. Add the cauliflower, zucchini, and bell pepper and cook for another 10 minutes, or until the vegetables are crisp-tender.

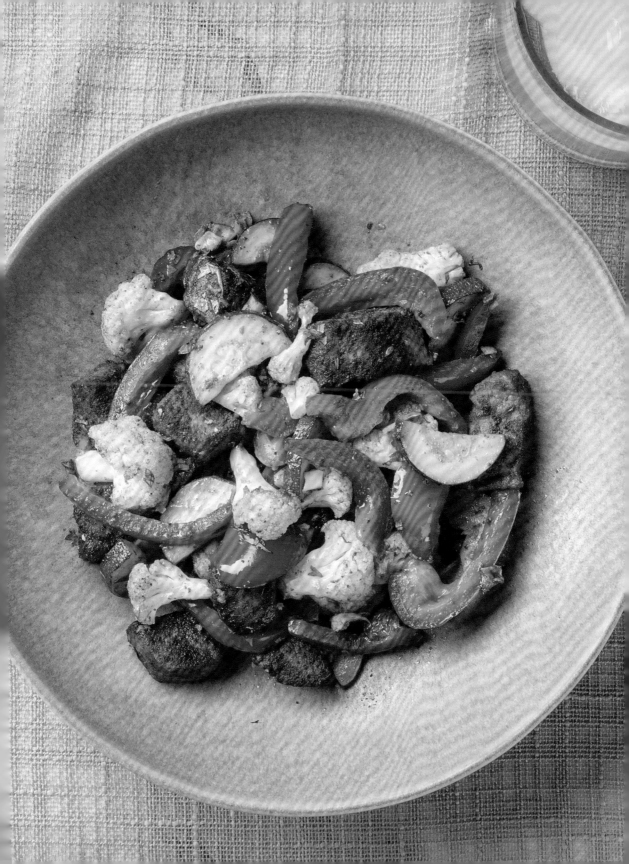

beef and mushroom
meatballs

italy

Raising three boys who were into hockey, basketball, lacrosse, swimming, and football, I knew they needed to fuel their intense activity with something hearty, otherwise my refrigerator would be raided constantly. Meatballs always did the trick. This recipe was sent from Metabolic Balance coaches in Italy and these tasty meatballs are great on a plate of spiralized zucchini (see the tip on page 169) or other vegetables.

Makes 1 serving

5 oz | 140 g beef tenderloin or beef fillet, ground (see note on page 191)

1 tbsp | 15 mL olive oil

1 large button mushroom, finely chopped

1 Roma tomato, finely chopped

½ onion, finely chopped

1 garlic clove, minced

1 tsp dried basil

Pinch dried oregano

Salt and black pepper to taste

Preheat the oven to 350°F | 175°C. Line a rimmed baking sheet with aluminum foil or parchment paper.

In a large bowl, mix the meat and the oil together, then add all of the other ingredients. Mix well and divide the mixture into 6 equal portions, then form each portion into a meatball.

Place the meatballs on the lined baking sheet. Bake until cooked through, about 20 minutes.

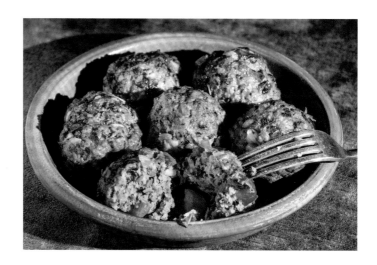

Special acknowledgment to Daniela Langellotti in Italy for this recipe.

heavenly
swedish meatballs

sweden

Thanks to the Metabolic Balance coaches in Sweden, these heavenly meatballs are easier to make than assembling IKEA flat-pack furniture. The meatballs don't require gravy; just serve on a bed of healthy red cabbage. The signature hint of allspice and nutmeg are comforting flavors and remind me of holidays with family.

Makes 4 servings

1 pound | 454 g beef tenderloin, ground (see note)

1 tbsp | 6 g rye flour

½ onion, finely chopped

¼ tsp ground nutmeg

¼ tsp ground allspice

¼ tsp finely chopped fresh parsley

Salt and black pepper to taste

1 tsp | 5 ml coconut oil or ghee

2 tbsp | 30 mL water

In a large bowl, combine the beef, flour, onion, nutmeg, allspice, parsley, and salt and pepper to taste and mix well. Let stand for 10 minutes, then form the mixture into about 24 small balls (about 2 tsp each).

Heat the oil in a large skillet over medium-high heat. Add the meatballs and fry them, stirring, until they have browned on all sides, 3–4 minutes. Add the water, reduce the heat to low, and cover the pan. Simmer the meatballs until cooked through, 6 minutes.

NOTE: Conventional ground beef is not included in Metabolic Balance plans because of the fat content. For recipes calling for ground beef tenderloin, I recommend buying a cut of tenderloin and having it ground (a butcher can do this for you). Divide it into single-serving portions and freeze any that you won't use within 1–2 days.

MAIN DISHES

Special acknowledgment to Susanna Rantala Ibsen in Sweden for this recipe.

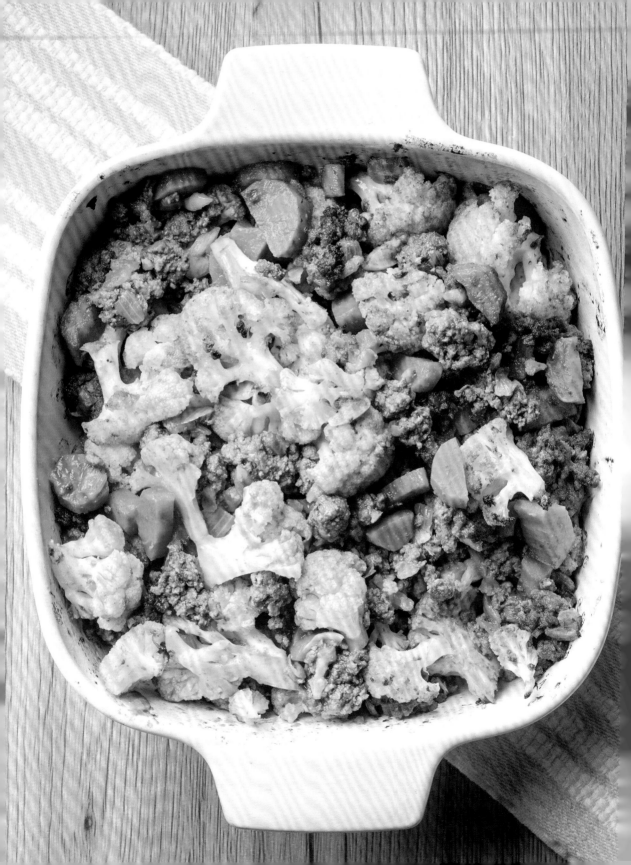

cauliflower casserole
with beef

As cauliflower grows, its coarse, ribbed leaves protect the head from sunlight, preventing the production of chlorophyll, which turns plants green. The result is the creamy white color. Cauliflower can also be purple or orange due to their phytochemical content, but the Metabolic Balance coaches in Turkey chose the traditional white for this casserole. The cooking process maintains the rich nutrients of the vegetables while keeping the beef tender.

Makes 2 servings

¼ cup | 60 mL olive oil

1 onion, finely chopped

10 oz | 285 g beef tenderloin, ground (see note on page 191)

1 tbsp | 15 g tomato paste

1 small head cauliflower, cut into small florets

2 medium carrots, sliced

2 tsp paprika

Salt and black pepper

1½ cups | 355 mL water

Preheat the broiler with a rack in the top third of the oven.

Heat the oil in a medium saucepan over medium-high heat. Add the onion and sauté until translucent, about 2 minutes.

Add the ground beef tenderloin, turn the heat down to medium, and cook until lightly browned, 7–10 minutes. Add the tomato paste and stir for 2 minutes, until thoroughly heated.

Add the cauliflower, carrots, paprika, and salt and pepper to taste and stir to coat with the ground beef mixture. Cover and cook for 5 minutes.

Add the water and cook for about 2 minutes, or until the cauliflower and carrots are crisp-tender and the mixture is hot. With a slotted spoon, transfer the mixture to a small casserole dish.

Broil on low until the top is browned, about 10 minutes.

Special acknowledgment to Sophie Kamuran Demirtas in Turkey for this recipe.

MAIN DISHES

crispy blackened salmon

I seek out the healthiest foods everywhere I travel. A wonderful meal I can find at our local restaurant, or as far away as Hong Kong, is blackened salmon. You don't need to leave home to enjoy this nutritious fish dish that is coated in spices and then pan-seared to perfection. Another fish that works well in this recipe is haddock, which, like salmon, is lower in mercury levels than many other fish. Serve with steamed or grilled vegetables of your choice, and rye crackers.

Makes 1 serving

½ tsp paprika

¼ tsp ground mustard

¼ tsp cayenne pepper

¼ tsp ground cumin

¼ tsp black pepper

¼ tsp white pepper

¼ tsp dried thyme

¼ tsp salt

1 tsp | 5 mL olive oil, divided

5 oz | 140 g salmon fillet

In a small bowl, combine the paprika, mustard, cayenne pepper, cumin, black pepper, white pepper, thyme, and salt; set aside.

Heat a cast iron skillet over high heat until extremely hot, 7–10 minutes.

Pour ½ tsp of the oil into a shallow plate. Dip the salmon fillet into the oil, turning to coat both sides. Sprinkle both sides with the spice mixture and gently pat mixture onto fish.

Place the fillet in the hot skillet. Carefully pour the remaining ½ tsp olive oil over the top of the fillet. Cook until the fish has a lightly charred appearance underneath, about 2 minutes. Turn the fillet over. Spoon the olive oil in the pan over the fish and cook until lightly charred on the other side, about 2 more minutes.

Why Vitamin D?

Take vitamin D daily while following the Metabolic Balance plan. Vitamin D is not only great for your bones, it is also a secret weapon to fight inflammation.

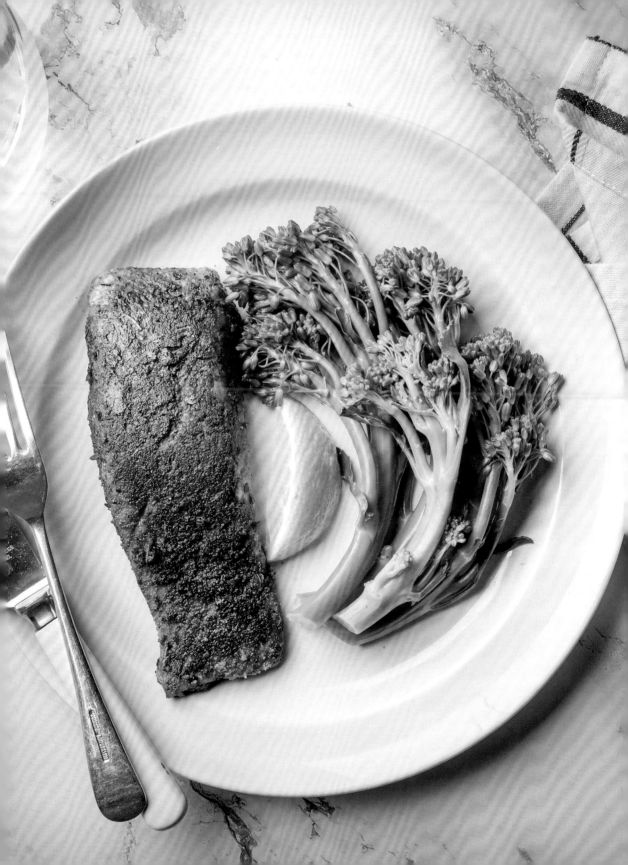

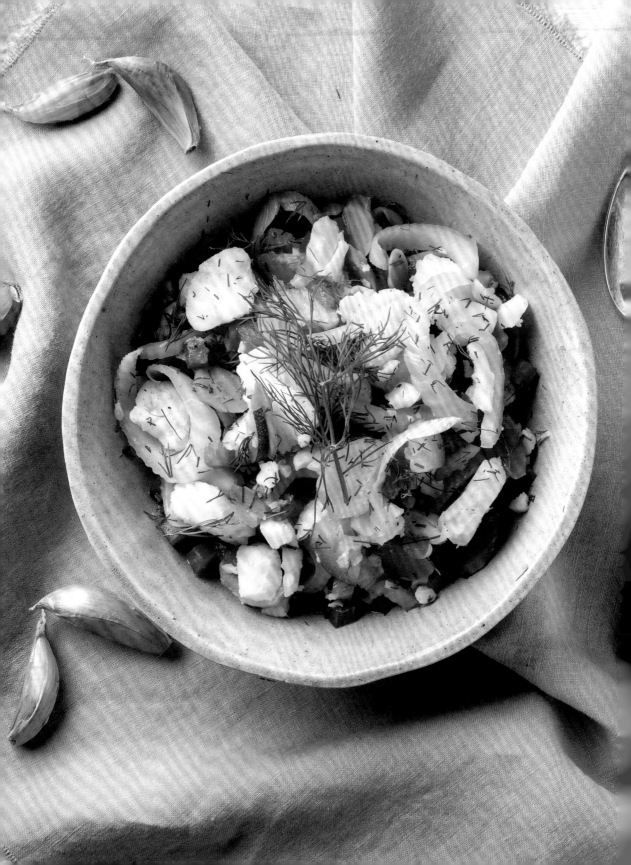

fragrant **fennel cod**

This fragrant stew is loaded with nutritious vegetables. It's delicious hot but just as good when eaten cold the next day, so it's a great choice for easy meal prep. Make a double batch and save yourself the cooking time the next day!

Makes 1 serving

5 oz | 140 g cod

1 cup | 90 g chopped fennel

½ cup | 100 g sliced zucchini

¼ cup | 40 g diced red bell pepper

1 small carrot, thinly sliced

1 small garlic clove, minced

¼ cup | 60 mL water

Salt and black pepper

Fennel frond, for garnish

Slice the cod into bite-size pieces. Set aside.

Combine the fennel, zucchini, bell pepper, carrot, garlic, and water in a medium saucepan. Cover and cook over medium heat for about 3 minutes to soften the vegetables.

Add the fish and cook for 3 minutes, or until the fish is cooked through and flaky. Stir everything together, season with salt and pepper to taste, and sprinkle with the fennel frond.

About the Ingredient: Fennel

One of fennel's unique phytonutrients, anethole, is the primary compound of its beneficial volatile oil and functions not only as an antioxidant but also as an anti-inflammatory compound.

spicy **scallop ceviche**

peru

While at a hot yoga retreat in Mexico, I took a cooking class in which I learned what some of you may already know: fish can be fully "cooked" without heat if soaked in fresh citrus juice. This traditional dish from the Metabolic Balance coaches in Peru tastes so clean and refreshing. Serve with a side salad, a cup of chopped mango, and a slice of rye bread or 2 rye crackers.

Makes 4 servings

1 pound | 454 g
sea scallops or cod or
other firm white fish

Juice of 7 limes

1 small red onion,
finely sliced

1 or 2 red chile peppers,
seeded and finely diced

2 tbsp chopped
fresh cilantro

1½ tsp salt

Cut the scallops or fish into ¾-in | 2-cm pieces.

In a medium bowl, combine the scallops, lime juice, onion, chiles, cilantro, and salt. Gently toss to incorporate everything. Cover with plastic wrap and refrigerate for 2 hours, but no longer or the fish will overcook.

Special acknowledgment to Deidad Vernal in Peru for this recipe.

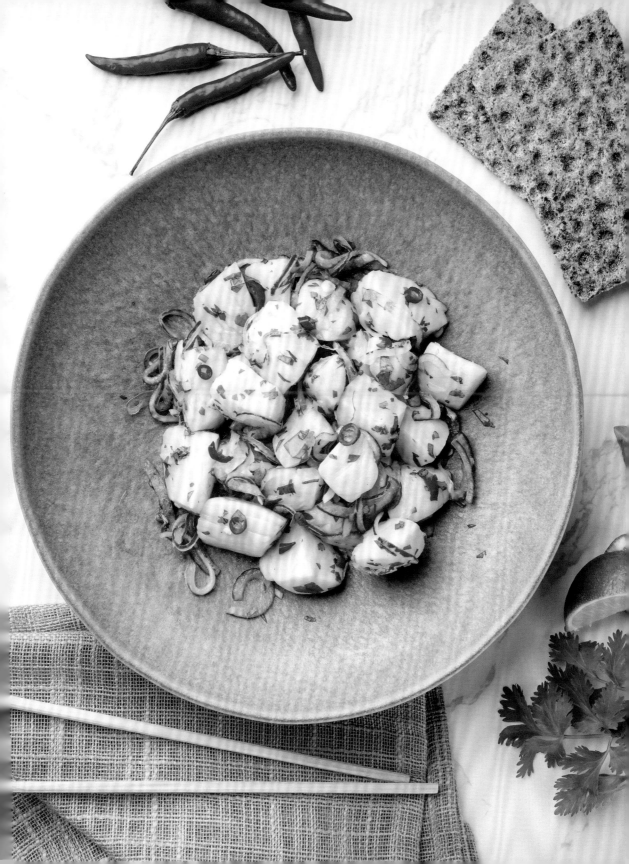

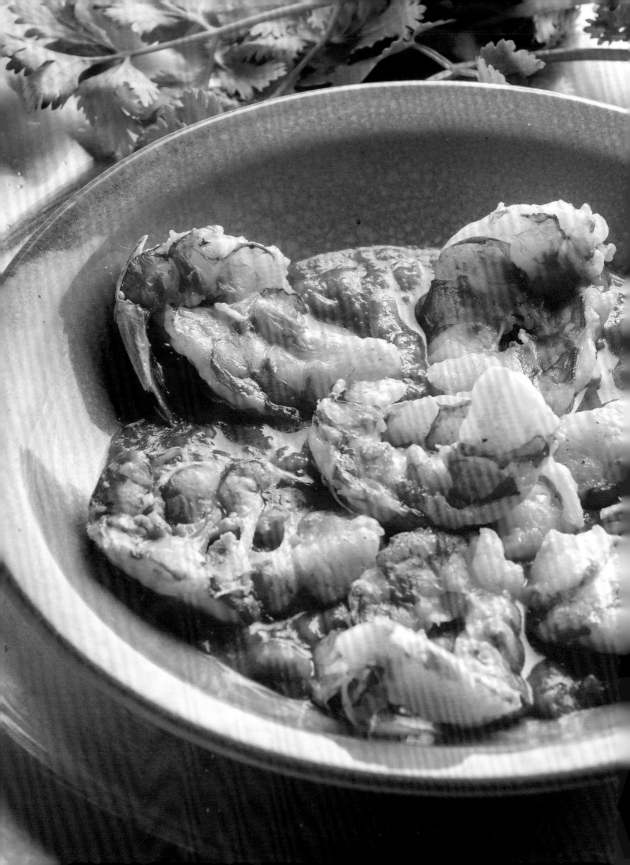

classic brazilian shrimp stew

Thank you, Metabolic Balance coaches from Brazil, for this classic shrimp dish. Fresh shrimp is ideal for this stew, although frozen will do. Just make sure you buy shrimp with the peels on in order to create the savory broth. The ingredient list is super simple, so this dish can be on your dinner table in about 35 minutes.

Makes 1 serving

5 oz | 140 g large shrimp, with shells and tails

1 garlic clove, peeled and cut into large pieces

⅓ red onion, cut into chunks

1 green onion, cut into large pieces

¼ tsp paprika

¼ tsp salt

¼ tsp black pepper

1½ cups | 355 mL water, or as needed

½ cup | 50 g cauliflower, cut into small pieces

⅓ medium carrot, diced

2 tsp | 10 mL ghee

Peel the shrimp, reserving the shells. Use a sharp knife to slit each shrimp down the back and remove the vein.

Put the shrimp shells and tails in a large pot, along with the garlic, red and green onions, paprika, salt, and pepper. Add enough water to cover.

Bring to a boil, then cover, reduce the heat, and simmer for 30 minutes. Set a strainer over a large bowl or another pot and strain the shrimp stock. Discard the solids and return the stock to the pot.

Add the cauliflower and carrot to the stock and cook over medium-high heat until tender, about 5 minutes.

Meanwhile, heat the ghee in a small skillet over medium-high heat. Fry the shrimp for 2 minutes on each side, until just cooked through. Take care not to overcook.

Using an immersion blender, blend the cauliflower and carrot mixture until it reaches your desired consistency, or transfer the mixture to a blender or food processor and puree, then return the puree to the pot.

Pour the puree into a bowl and add the cooked shrimp.

Special acknowledgment to Melissa Pancini in Brazil for this recipe.

MAIN DISHES

prawns on the barbie
with grilled asparagus

I love the smell of prawns (shrimp) cooking on the grill. It makes me think of parties and extravagance, and I know that it's going to be a joy to eat. This dish from the Metabolic Balance coaches in Australia is so simple I've added it to my regular meal rotation. Rosemary is a pleasant surprise, something I never would have thought to add to shrimp. If you prefer, you can serve the shrimp with salad greens instead of the grilled asparagus. When preparing the shrimp, leave the shells on as this protects the meat from the heat and adds to the flavor.

Makes 2 servings

10 oz | 285 g medium or large shrimp or prawns

3 tbsp | 45 mL olive oil, divided

1 tsp finely chopped fresh rosemary

4 garlic cloves, minced

1 tsp finely grated lemon zest

2 tsp | 10 mL apple cider vinegar or fresh lemon juice

Salt and black pepper

1 bunch asparagus, ends trimmed

Use a sharp knife to slit each shrimp down the back and remove the vein (leave the shells on).

Put the shrimp in a bowl and add 1 tbsp of the olive oil, the rosemary, garlic, lemon zest, vinegar, and salt and pepper to taste. Gently toss to coat and set aside to marinate for 20 minutes.

Meanwhile, preheat the grill.

Toss the asparagus in 1 tbsp of the remaining olive oil and place on the grill, perpendicular to the grate. Cook for 1 minute, then roll the asparagus around to cook on all sides, another 1–2 minutes. Transfer to a plate.

Lay the shrimp on the grill shell-side down. Cook for 3 minutes, or until shrimp turn from translucent to white and become opaque. Turn them over and cook for another minute.

Transfer the shrimp to a plate and drizzle with the remaining 1 tbsp olive oil. Serve immediately.

Special acknowledgment to Zita Dixon in Australia for this recipe.

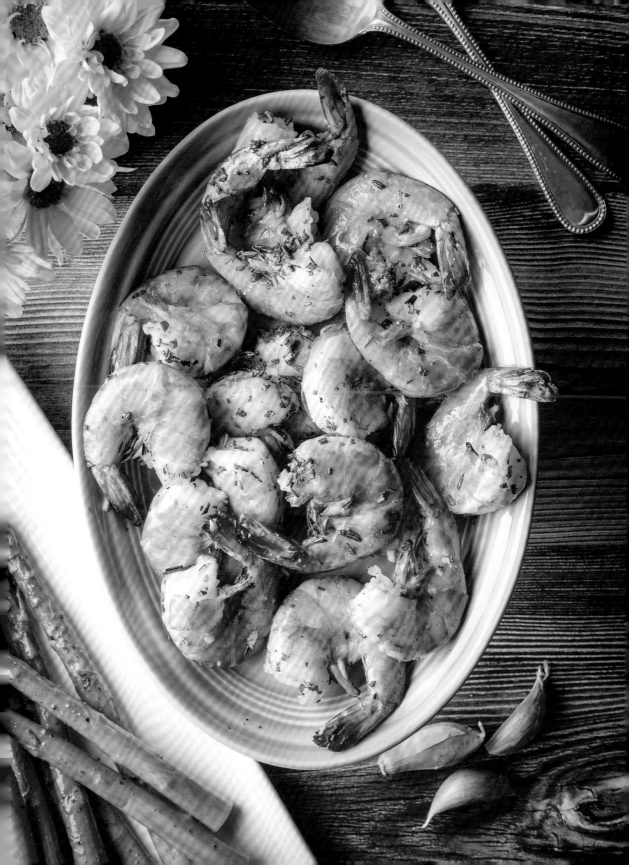

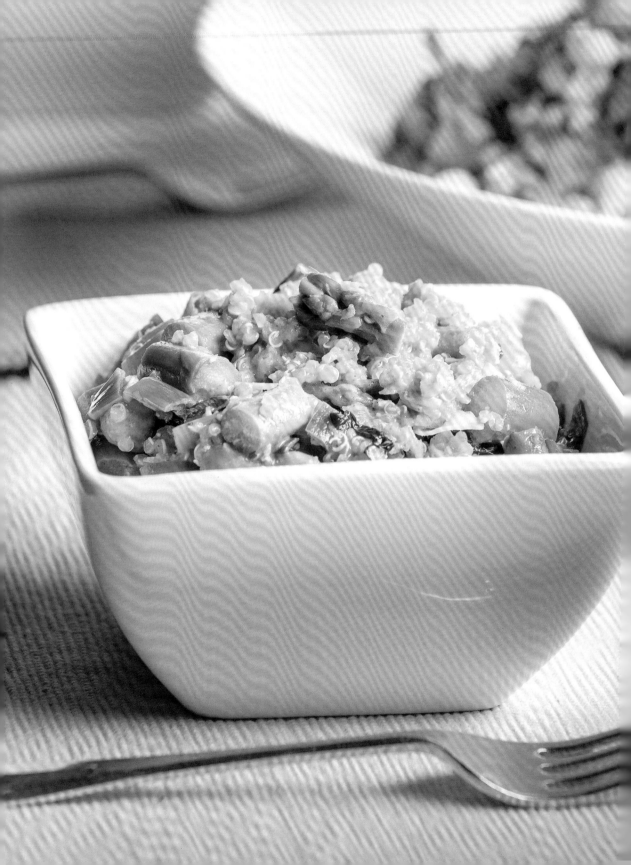

spicy coconut curry quinoa
with chickpeas

treat meal

I once visited an Ayurvedic spa in India that served a dish like this, and I ate it every day while I was there. When I returned home, I could hardly wait to re-create it in my kitchen. It's a great dish for a family, as this recipe makes 4 servings.

Makes 4 servings

3 cups | 710 mL water

1½ cups | 250 g uncooked quinoa

2 bunches asparagus, ends trimmed

5 tbsp | 75 mL coconut oil

3–4 heaping tbsp | 45–60 mL red curry paste, mild, medium or hot (to taste)

2 bunches green onions, sliced diagonally

2 pounds | 900 g baby spinach

2 cups | 475 mL coconut milk

4 cups | 560 g canned cooked chickpeas, drained and rinsed

1 cup | 60 g unsweetened shredded coconut

Salt and black pepper

In a medium saucepan, bring the water to a boil. Add the quinoa, cover, turn the heat down to low, and cook for 15 minutes, or until the water is absorbed and the quinoa is tender. Remove from the heat.

Meanwhile, fill a large pot with water and bring to a boil. Add the asparagus and cook for 2 minutes to blanch it. Using tongs, transfer the asparagus to a cutting board and let cool slightly. When cool enough to handle, cut into bite-size pieces. Set aside.

Heat the oil in a large skillet or wok over medium-high heat. Add the curry paste and green onions and stir until the onions are coated in the paste and wilted, 1–2 minutes. Working in batches as necessary, stir in the spinach and sauté until wilted, about 6 minutes total.

Add the coconut milk, chickpeas, quinoa, and asparagus. Turn the heat down to low, cover, and simmer, stirring frequently, for 10 minutes to heat thoroughly. Stir in the shredded coconut. Season with salt and pepper to taste.

TIP: Not all prepared curry pastes are the same. Some are saltier than others. Make sure you taste the dish and adjust the seasoning according to your taste.

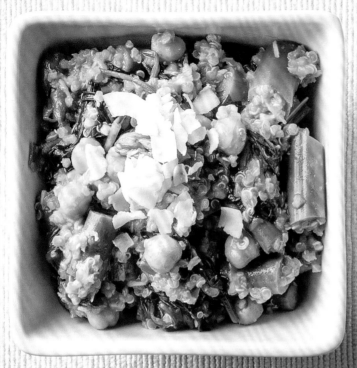
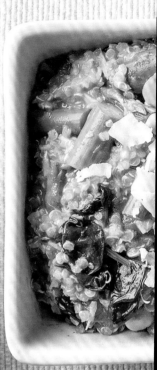

If possible, do not eat after 9:00 pm.

Not eating between 9:00 pm and the following morning allows for an overnight fast. Studies show that when you eat after dinner, your body will store those calories as fat and you will gain weight rather than burning the food as energy. Fasting will also train your body to become more efficient at burning fat. Eating at night also prevents your body from powering down, as digestion requires a tremendous amount of energy. Fasting overnight also allows you to sleep better, and you will wake up feeling more energized.

See pages 34, 39, 60, 65, and 131 for the other Rules of Metabolic Balance!

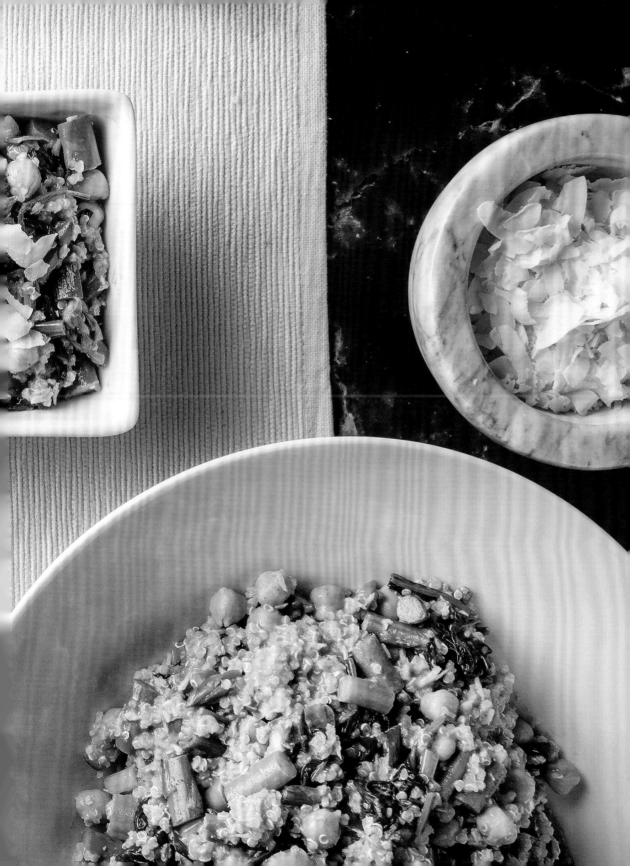

tofu vegetable stir-fry

Tofu contains several anti-inflammatory, antioxidant phytochemicals, making it a great addition to an anti-inflammatory diet. Tofu is versatile, particularly because on its own it has a creamy, neutral taste and absorbs the delicious flavors of whatever it is cooked with. This dish has a lot of flavor and is easy to prepare.

Makes 1 serving

3 oz | 85 g firm tofu

1 tbsp | 15 mL olive oil

¼ tsp coriander seeds

¼ tsp mustard seeds

½ yellow onion, cut into small dice

⅔ cup | 50 g broccoli florets

¼ red bell pepper, diced

1 button mushroom, diced

⅛ tsp ground cardamom

Salt and black pepper

Press the tofu to remove excess liquid and improve its texture: Put a paper towel on a plate and place the tofu on top. Cover with another paper towel and another plate. Place something heavy on top to weigh it down, like a few books or a can of tomatoes, to press out the extra liquid. Leave the tofu for 15 minutes, changing paper towels if needed. Cut the tofu into 1-in | 2.5-cm cubes or rectangles and set aside.

Heat the oil in a large skillet over medium-high heat. Add the coriander seeds and mustard seeds and cook for 30–60 seconds, until the mustard seeds start to pop. Add the onion and sauté for 2 minutes, tossing to coat. Add the broccoli, bell pepper, and mushroom and stir-fry for 5–7 minutes, until the vegetables are softened.

Add the cardamom and tofu and stir to coat. Stir-fry for 3–5 minutes until the vegetables are crisp-tender. Season with salt and pepper to taste.

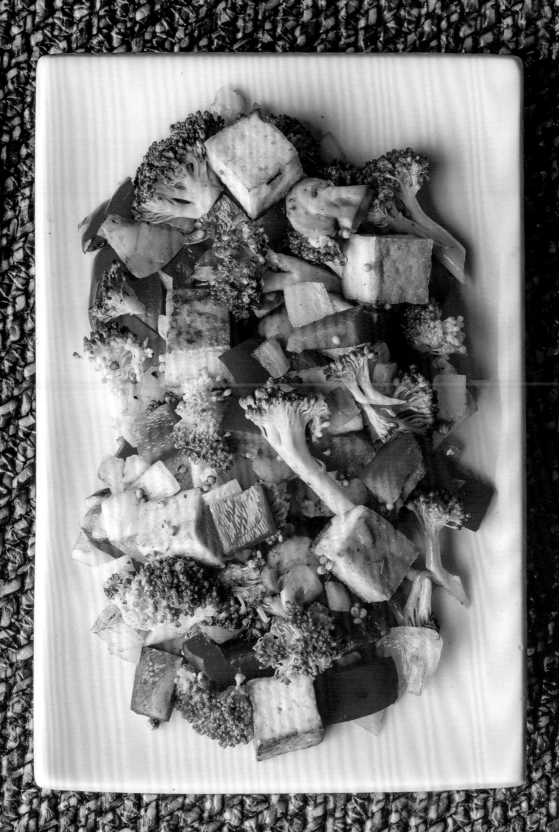

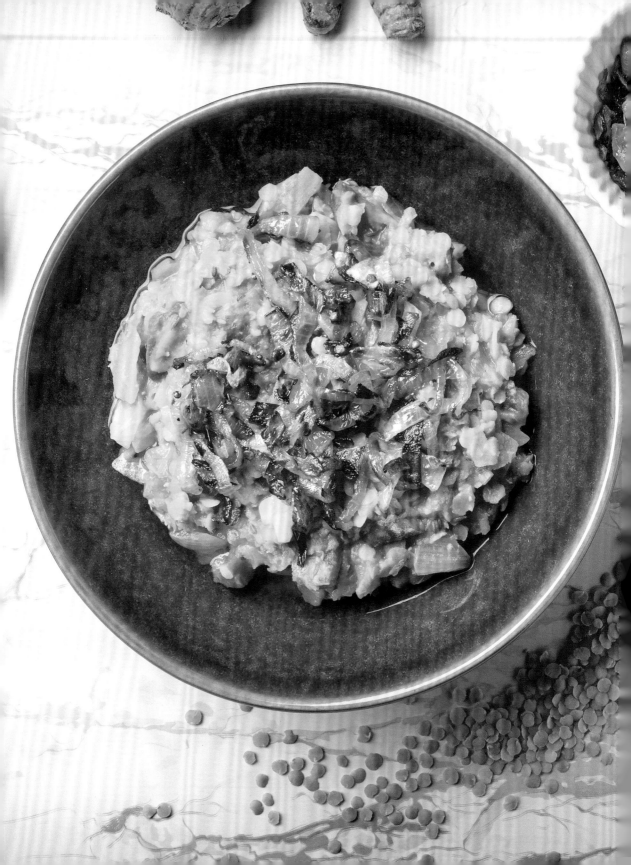

flavorful **tadka dal**

Because I have come to love exercise so much, I have a big appetite. Often, I can eat more than my grown sons, and Metabolic Balance recipes help me stay fit and feel satiated. This dish from the Metabolic Balance coaches in India is so thick, dense, and satisfying, it is the perfect meal after a workout. I like it hot and often increase the spices. Serve it with a slice of rye bread.

Makes 1 serving

¼ cup | 60 g dry red lentils, rinsed and drained

1 large tomato, chopped

1 onion, half finely chopped and half thinly sliced, divided

1 garlic clove, finely chopped

1 (1-in | 2.5-cm) piece fresh ginger, minced

1 tsp ground cumin

½ tsp ground turmeric

½ tsp salt, or more to taste

¼ tsp curry powder, or more to taste

1 cup | 240 mL water

¼ tsp red pepper flakes

In a medium pot, combine the lentils, tomato, chopped onion, garlic, ginger, cumin, turmeric, salt, curry powder, and water and bring to a boil over high heat. Reduce the heat to medium, partially cover, and cook for 10–15 minutes, stirring occasionally, until the lentils are tender.

Meanwhile, heat a small nonstick skillet over medium heat. Add the sliced onion and red pepper flakes and sauté until the onion is softened and the edges are lightly browned, 4–5 minutes.

Stir the lentils vigorously to make a creamy consistency, adding a little water if they are too thick or cooking for a few minutes with the lid off if they are too runny.

Check the seasoning of the lentils and add additional salt and curry powder as needed. Top the lentils with the browned onion.

Special acknowledgment to Taranjeet Kaur in India for this recipe.

MAIN DISHES

south asian **tofu**

india

Regular intake of soy protein can help lower total cholesterol levels by up to 30 percent, is anti-inflammatory, has antioxidant properties, and is considered heart healthy. The Metabolic Balance coaches in India sent this local dish featuring tofu. It's delicious and has a bit of bite from the red pepper flakes. It's light and refreshing and I enjoy it with rye bread or rye chapati.

Makes 1 serving

3 oz | 85 g firm tofu

1 tbsp | 15 mL ghee

¼ tsp mustard seeds

½ carrot, cut into matchsticks

¼ green bell pepper, thinly sliced

6 baby bok choy leaves, sliced

3 curry leaves
or fresh basil leaves

¼ tsp salt

¼ tsp red pepper flakes

Pinch ground turmeric

Press the tofu to remove excess liquid and improve its texture: Put a paper towel on a plate and place the tofu on top. Cover with another paper towel and another plate. Place something heavy on top to weigh it down, like a few books or a can of tomatoes, to press out the extra liquid. Leave the tofu for 15 minutes, changing paper towels if needed. Cut the tofu into 1-in | 2.5-cm cubes and set aside.

Heat the ghee in a medium skillet over medium heat. Add the mustard seeds and let them sputter for a few seconds so they release their flavor. Add the carrot, bell pepper, bok choy, and curry leaves and stir-fry for 1 minute to soften. Add the tofu, salt, red pepper flakes, and turmeric and stir to coat the tofu and vegetables in the spices.

Cover, reduce the heat to medium-low, and cook for 3–4 minutes, until the vegetables are softened. Stir and serve hot.

About the Ingredient: Tofu

Tofu is also known as bean curd. It is a highly nutritious, protein-rich food made from soybeans. It is full of important nutrients like selenium, magnesium, calcium, and omega-3 fatty acids. Tofu has very little flavor on its own but will absorb the delicious flavors of other foods and seasonings, which makes it adaptable to many recipes.

Special acknowledgment to Taranjeet Kaur in India for this recipe.

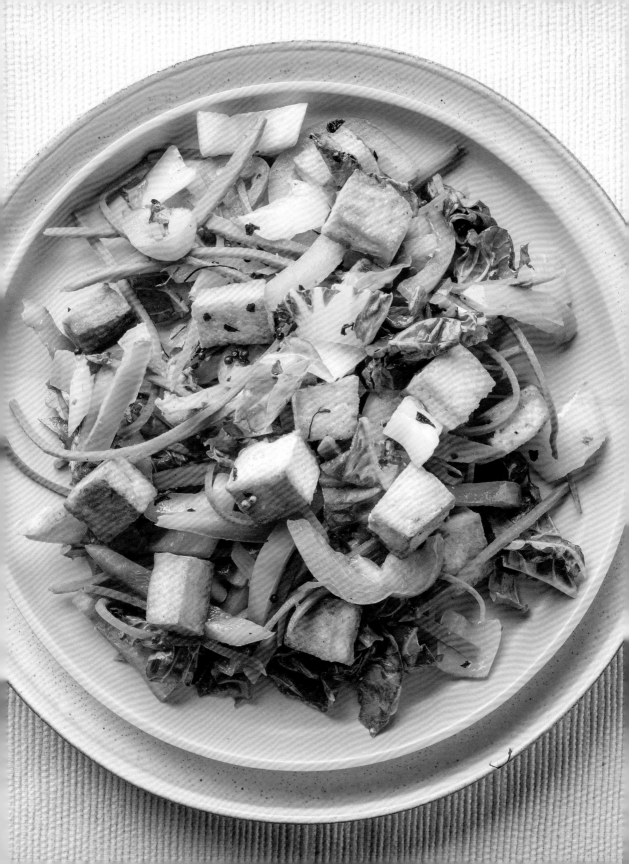

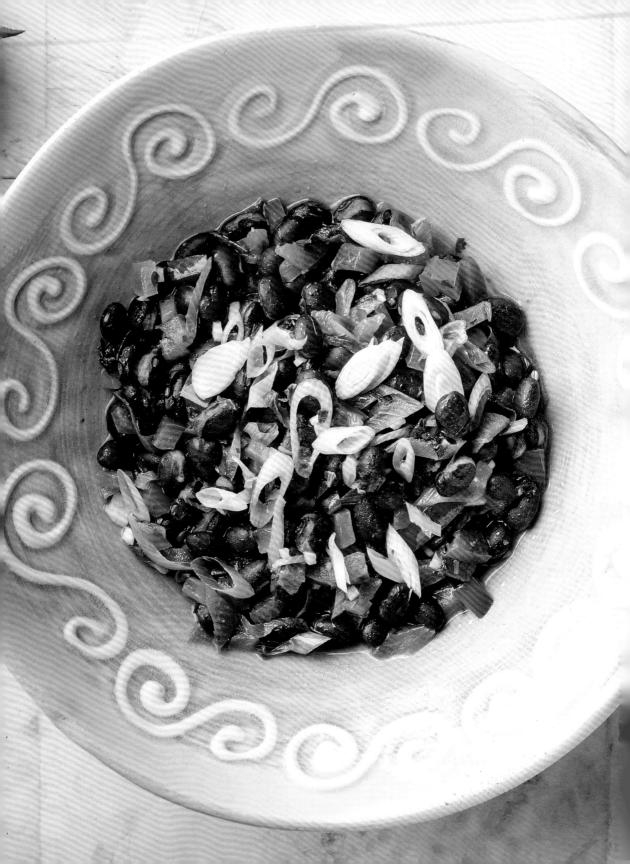

feijoada **bean stew**

brazil

Beans are the culinary symbol of Brazil, and Brazilians typically eat them at least once a day. Black beans are loaded with fiber and are a great source of tryptophan, which promotes relaxation. This flavorful bean stew shared by the Metabolic Balance coaches in Brazil will surely stick to your ribs, but with a feeling of lightness. Enjoy it with rye bread for a full meal.

Makes 1 serving

1 tbsp | 15 mL ghee

1 garlic clove, minced

2 tbsp | 20 g chopped red onion

1 green onion, chopped

¼ red bell pepper, diced

2 tbsp chopped fresh parsley

2 tbsp chopped fresh cilantro

¾ cup | 130 g canned black beans, drained and rinsed

⅛ tsp ground cumin

⅛ tsp paprika

¼ cup | 60 mL water

Special acknowledgment to Melissa Pancini in Brazil for this recipe.

Heat the ghee in a medium pot over medium-low heat. Add the garlic, red and green onions, bell pepper, parsley, and cilantro and sauté for about 5 minutes, or until the bell pepper is softened. Add the black beans, cumin, paprika, and water and stir. Turn the heat down to low and cook, stirring occasionally, until the liquid thickens, about 15 minutes.

Exercise on the Metabolic Balance Program

Exercise has many benefits. It releases the feel-good hormone serotonin, builds muscle mass, and boosts confidence. It is the ultimate healer because it helps you get what your body wants: oxygen. Oxygen is the fuel that feeds every cell in your body. When you move, you pump oxygen through your veins and that is how you gain strength and energy and feel amazing. Getting enough oxygen gives you the emotional and physical strength to overcome depression, anxiety, and fatigue, and heal from injuries.

Any type of activity that you enjoy doing is great, and you don't have to go to the gym. I encourage my clients to achieve a total of 1 hour a day of exercise, and it does not have to be at one time. It all adds up to your increased health and happiness and can be as simple as taking the stairs instead of the elevator, parking farther away than necessary, and getting up from your desk frequently to take short walks.

roasted chickpeas and vegetables

Roasting brings out the natural sugars of vegetables, releasing aromatic compounds that offer up a feast of flavors. Roasting chickpeas, also known as garbanzo beans, gives them a satisfying, crispy texture. This tasty plant-based meal is affordable, and also rich in fiber and protein.

Makes 2 servings

2 cups | 330 g
canned chickpeas,
rinsed and drained

½ red onion,
cut into chunks

½ cup | 50 g
cauliflower florets

½ carrot, cut into chunks

½ orange bell pepper,
cut into chunks

2 tbsp | 30 mL olive oil

½ tsp dried
herbes de Provence

Preheat the oven to 450°F | 230°C.

Combine the chickpeas, onion, cauliflower, carrot, and bell pepper in a small baking dish. Drizzle the oil over the vegetables and chickpeas, add the herbes de Provence, and toss.

Roast, stirring every 5 minutes, until the vegetables are tender and lightly browned and the chickpeas are crispy, about 20 minutes.

TIP: This dish is best enjoyed right after making it, because the chickpeas will lose their crispiness if stored.

Why Chewing Matters

Chewing food well is essential for proper digestion. The enzyme amylase is released in your saliva when food is chewed well. Amylase begins to break down carbohydrates in the mouth, which then enables food to be digested with greater ease. Chewing also allows food particles to be small enough for the gastric juices to degrade them and make more nutrients available for absorption. Chewing slowly and thoroughly also helps prevent overeating.

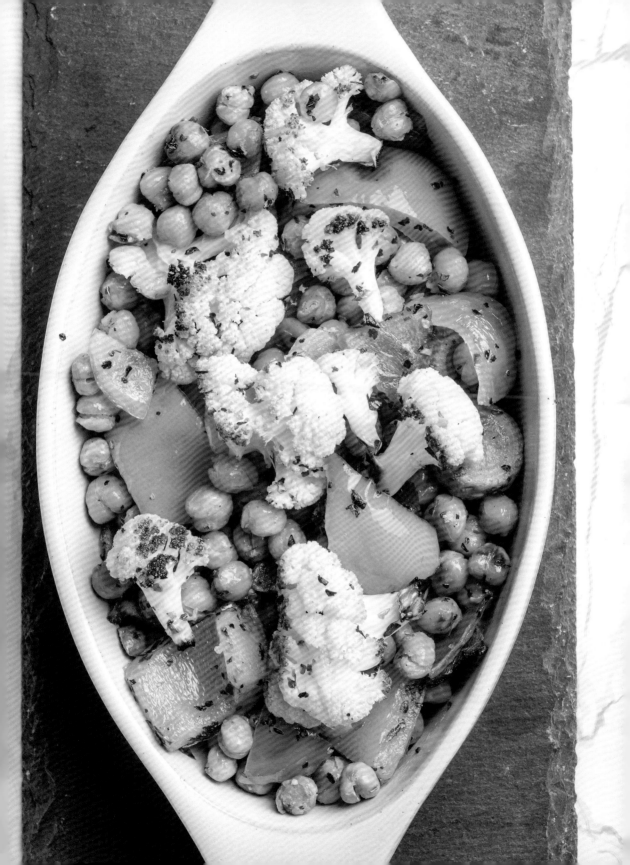

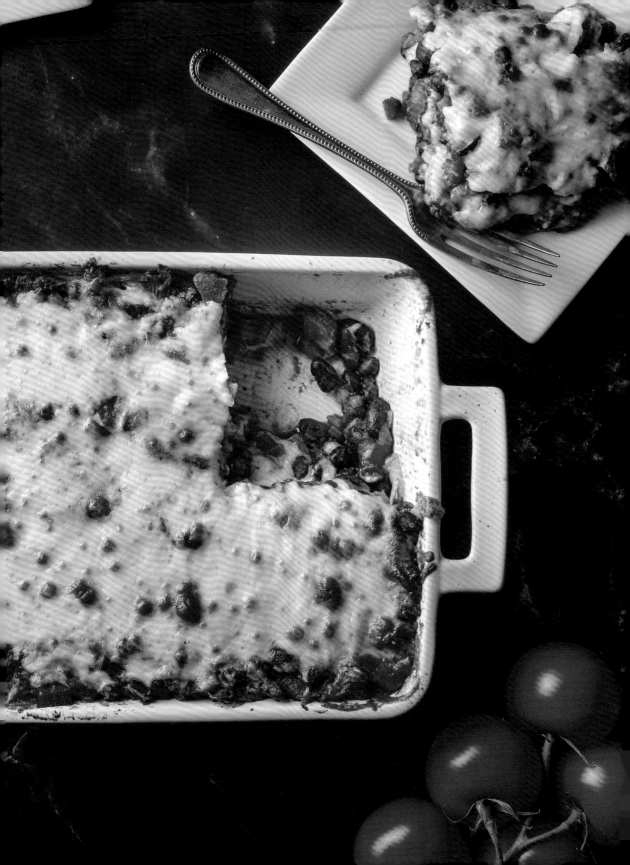

two-bean **tortilla lasagna**

treat meal

My friend Todd came to visit our family at our lake cottage one summer and brought a giant pan of this fabulous Tex Mex–inspired lasagna. Everyone was shocked that it was meatless and noodle-free! It takes just minutes to prepare and once in the oven, the aromas become increasingly enticing. Serve with a green salad on the side.

Makes 6–8 servings

1 tbsp butter

2 tbsp | 30 mL olive oil

2 medium yellow onions, diced

2 garlic cloves, minced

1½ red bell peppers, diced

1 (28-oz | 794-g) can diced tomatoes, undrained

2 cups | 360 g canned black beans, drained

2 cups | 360 g canned kidney beans, drained

1 cup | 240 mL mild or medium salsa

2 tbsp ground cumin

4 soft multigrain (approximately 12 in | 30 cm) or 8 soft corn (approximately 6 in | 15 cm) tortillas

3⅓ cups | 400 g grated Monterey Jack cheese

Sliced green onion, for garnish (optional)

Preheat the oven to 350°F | 175°C. Grease a 9 x 13-in | 33 x 23 cm casserole dish or baking pan with the butter.

Heat the oil in a large skillet over medium heat. Add the onions, garlic, and bell peppers and sauté until softened, or about 3 minutes. Stir in the tomatoes with their juices, black beans, kidney beans, salsa, and cumin. Simmer the bean mixture until heated through, 10–15 minutes.

In the prepared casserole dish, layer one-third of the bean mix, then 2 tortillas, then half of the remaining bean mix, then half of the cheese. Cover with the remaining 2 tortillas, the remaining bean mix, and the remaining cheese.

Place the casserole dish on a rimmed baking sheet to catch drips and bake for 45 minutes, or until the bean mix is bubbling and the cheese is lightly browned. Sprinkle with the green onion.

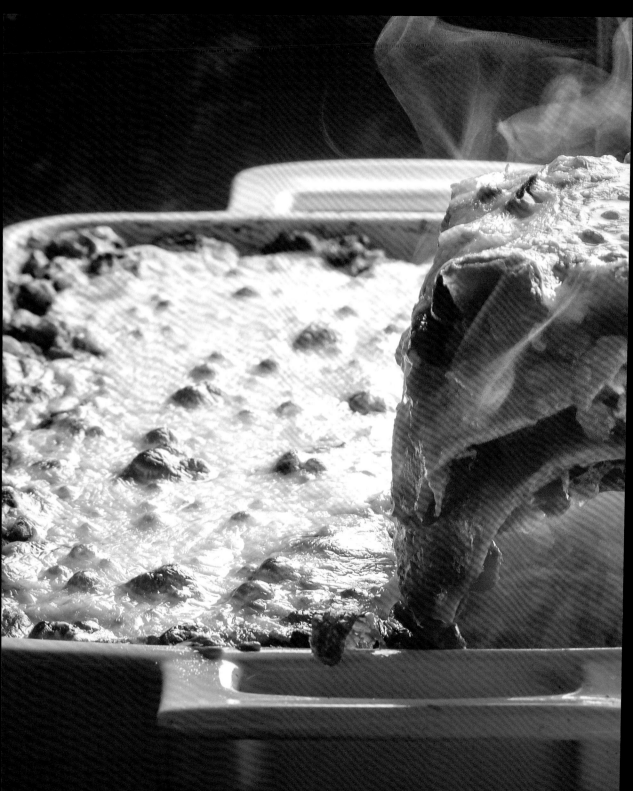

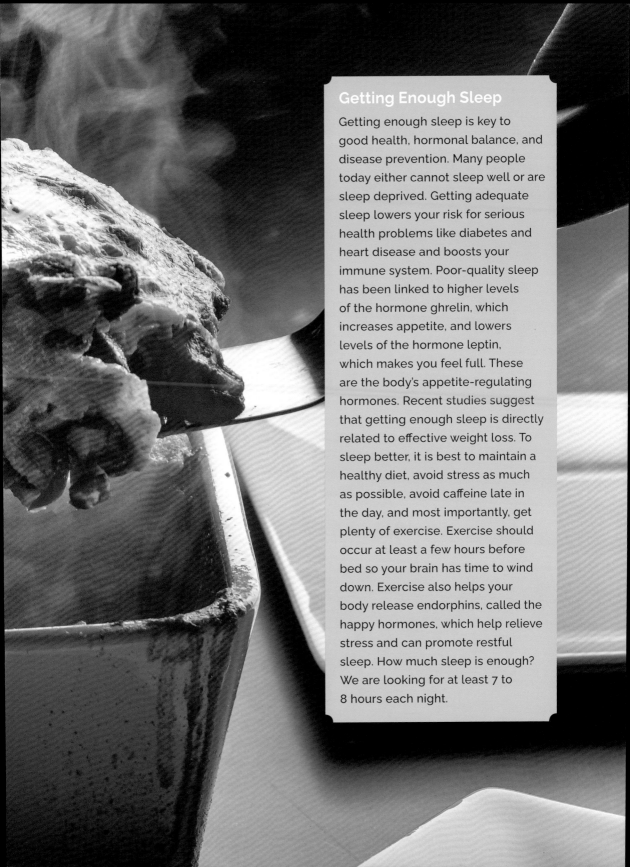

Getting Enough Sleep

Getting enough sleep is key to good health, hormonal balance, and disease prevention. Many people today either cannot sleep well or are sleep deprived. Getting adequate sleep lowers your risk for serious health problems like diabetes and heart disease and boosts your immune system. Poor-quality sleep has been linked to higher levels of the hormone ghrelin, which increases appetite, and lowers levels of the hormone leptin, which makes you feel full. These are the body's appetite-regulating hormones. Recent studies suggest that getting enough sleep is directly related to effective weight loss. To sleep better, it is best to maintain a healthy diet, avoid stress as much as possible, avoid caffeine late in the day, and most importantly, get plenty of exercise. Exercise should occur at least a few hours before bed so your brain has time to wind down. Exercise also helps your body release endorphins, called the happy hormones, which help relieve stress and can promote restful sleep. How much sleep is enough? We are looking for at least 7 to 8 hours each night.

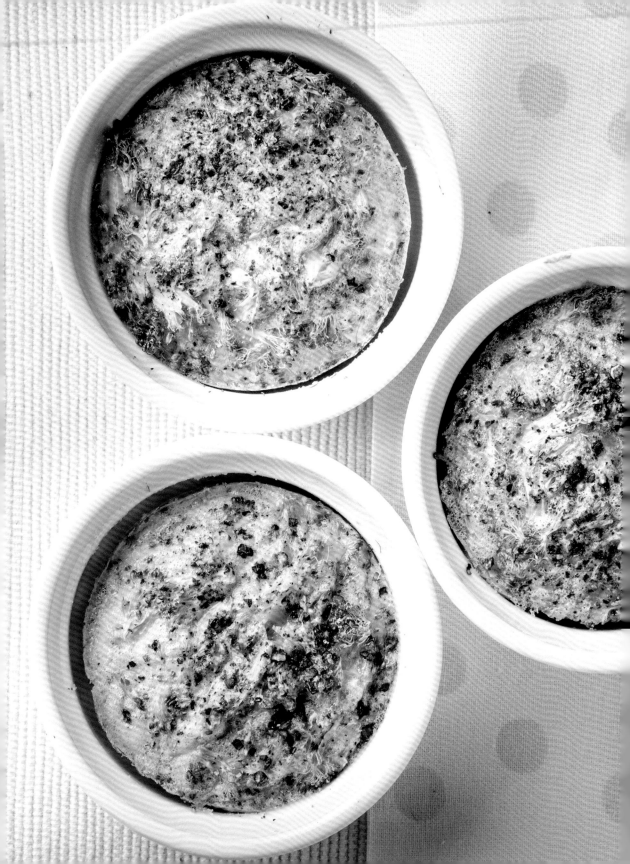

easy **broccoli soufflés**

italy

Before I learned to make soufflés, I thought they required special culinary skills. The Metabolic Balance coaches in Italy assured me of the simplicity of this recipe. The fragrant taste of nutmeg brings a surprising element to this light, airy dish that is reminiscent of a caffè (coffee) in Rome. For a full meal, enjoy your soufflés with a salad, rye crackers, and a serving of fresh papaya.

Makes 1 serving

2 large eggs

⅛ tsp ground nutmeg

Salt and black pepper

1¼ cups | 120 g broccoli florets

Preheat the oven to 350°F | 175°C.

In a medium bowl, whisk together the eggs, nutmeg, and salt and pepper to taste. Set aside.

Bring a small saucepan of water to a boil. Add the broccoli and blanch for 2 minutes. Drain, pouring the hot water into a baking dish to a depth of about 1 in | 2.5 cm to make a water bath for baking. Set aside.

Blitz the broccoli in a food processor until smooth. Stir it gently into the eggs.

Divide the mixture evenly between 2 small ramekins. Place the ramekins in the water bath. Cover the ramekins lightly with aluminum foil.

Bake for 20 minutes, or until the soufflés have set and risen. Carefully lift the foil. The eggs shouldn't jiggle if you wiggle the dish.

Special acknowledgment to Daniela Langellotti in Italy for this recipe.

MAIN DISHES

mirza ghasemi (roasted eggplant and tomato)

iran

Our Metabolic Balance coaches in Iran sent us this delightful dinner twist. This tasty dish is made of eggplant and tomato held together with eggs. The roasted eggplant makes the whole dish creamy. Mirza Ghasemi is often served as an appetizer, but pair it with Metabolic Balance–friendly wild rice, and it makes a delightful dinner. Eggplant is a great source of fiber, available in a rainbow of colors, from lavender to jade green, orange, and yellow-white.

Makes 1 serving

1 tsp butter

½ medium eggplant, halved lengthwise

1 tbsp | 15 mL coconut oil

½ medium tomato, chopped

2 garlic cloves, minced

½ tsp salt

⅛ tsp ground turmeric

Pinch black pepper

2 large eggs, lightly beaten

Preheat the broiler with a rack in the top third of the oven.

Grease a rimmed baking sheet with butter and place the eggplant skin side up on the pan and broil until the skin is blistered, about 3 minutes. Using tongs, turn the eggplant over and broil until the flesh is soft, about 3 minutes. The timing will depend on how hot and close the boiler is, so keep an eye on the eggplant to make sure it doesn't burn.

Transfer the eggplant to a cutting board to cool slightly. When it is cool enough to handle, remove and discard the skin. Cut the eggplant flesh into cubes.

Heat the coconut oil in a nonstick skillet over medium heat. Add the eggplant, tomato, garlic, salt, turmeric, and pepper and stir-fry for 2 minutes to soften the tomato and release the flavors from the garlic and turmeric. Add the eggs and stir until eggs are cooked through, 2–4 minutes.

Special acknowledgment to Couros Kamal in Iran for this recipe.

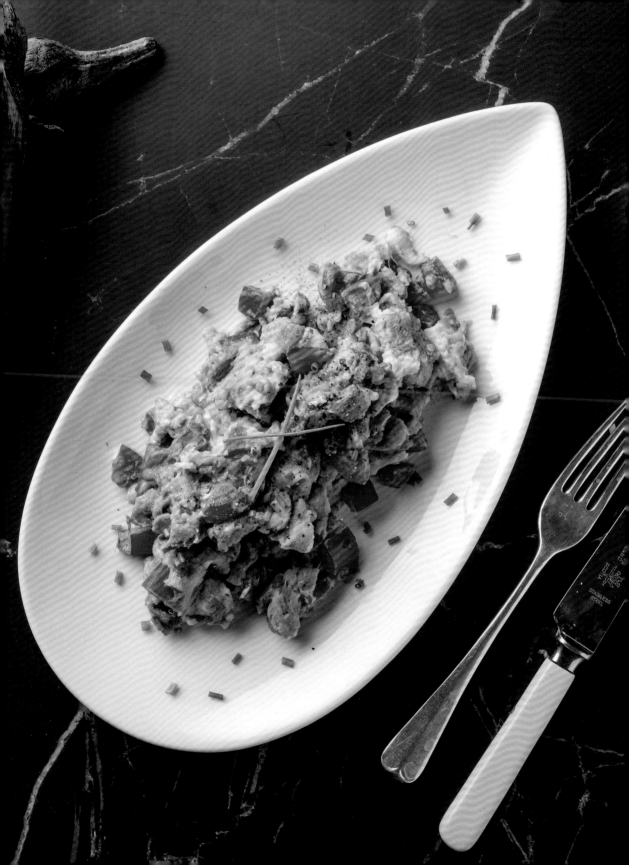

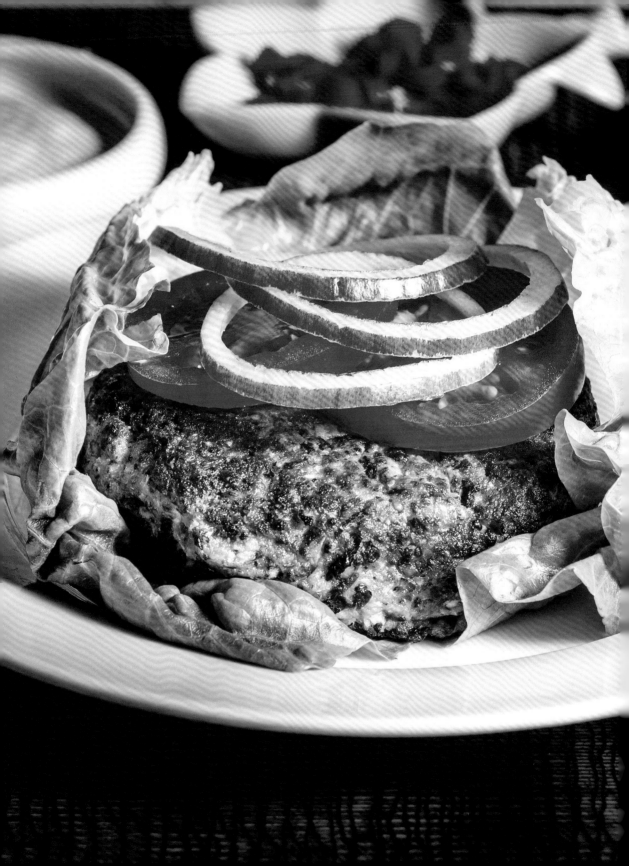

light black bean burgers

Before a hot yoga class after work, I prefer to have eaten a lighter lunch. This burger gives me the comfort that a regular burger would provide but without the heaviness. Serve on lettuce with tomato and red onion slices. They're also good with a squirt of fresh lemon juice.

Makes 2 servings

1¾ cups | 300 g canned black beans, drained and rinsed

½ small zucchini, chopped

2 tbsp chopped onion

2 rye crackers (such as Wasa or Ryvita)

¼ tsp garlic powder

Salt and black pepper

1 tbsp | 15 mL coconut oil

In a food processor, combine the beans, zucchini, onion, crackers, garlic powder, and salt and pepper to taste. Pulse the mixture until just combined and sticky; do not puree. Divide the mixture in half, then shape each portion into a patty about 1 in | 2.5 cm thick.

Heat the oil in a medium skillet over high heat. Cook the patties for 5–7 minutes on each side, until browned.

sautéed mushroom and vegetable delight

This colorful dish is simple to prepare and provides powerful nutrition. I love the crunch of the veggies, along with the meaty texture of the mushrooms. This is a surprisingly filling recipe that you can enjoy for lunch or dinner.

Makes 1 serving

5¼ oz | 150 g shiitake or oyster mushrooms

1 tbsp | 15 mL olive oil

1 small garlic clove, minced

1 (1-in | 2.5-cm) piece ginger, grated

1 medium carrot, cut into ½-in | 1.25-cm pieces

¼ cup | 40 g chopped red and/or orange bell pepper

½ cup | 115 g chopped cabbage

1 tsp dried oregano

Salt and black pepper

½ cup | 120 mL vegetable broth

1 green onion, sliced diagonally

Clean any dirt off the mushrooms with a paper towel or the edge of a knife, but don't wash them with water. Thinly slice the mushrooms. Set aside.

Heat the oil in a medium skillet over medium heat. Add the garlic and ginger and sauté for 1 minute. Add the carrot, bell pepper, cabbage, oregano, and salt and pepper to taste and sauté for 5 minutes. Stir in the broth. Add the green onion and mushrooms and cook until the mushrooms are soft, 5–7 minutes.

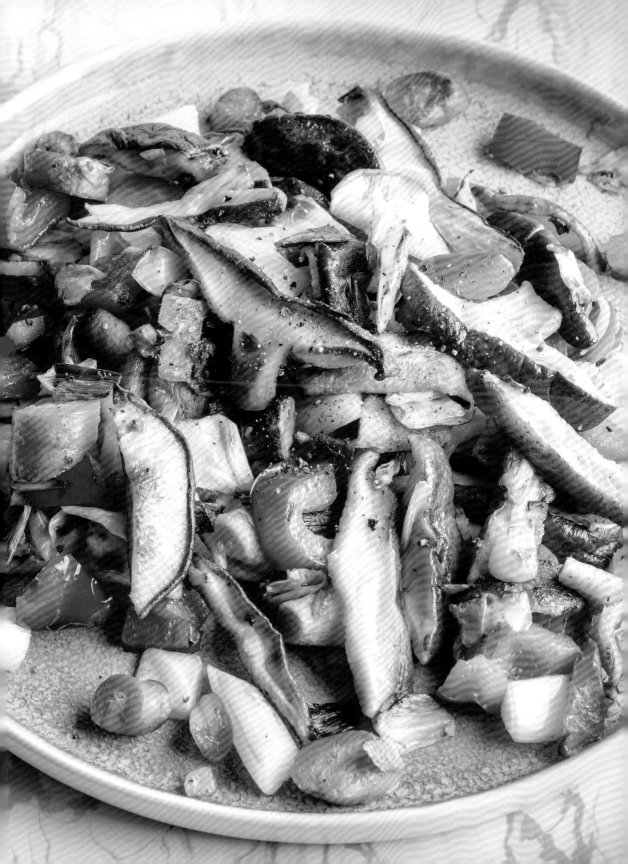

Acknowledgments

The largest thanks goes to my editor and agent, Anne Archer Butcher, who has also been my mentor and marketing coach for decades. Thank you for believing in me and taking me on a journey to manifest my dreams. I am so grateful for everything you have done for me. This book could not have happened without your incredible inspiration and support. Thank you for pushing me to excellence and guiding me each step of the way.

Thank you to Amanda Fitzgibbon, my personal assistant, for your patience and guidance. It has been a total joy to work with you over the years. Thank you also to Fiona Jones, who helped test every recipe and kept me totally organized.

Thank you to Claire Schulz at BenBella Books for her wonderful professional and editorial support. She helped guide every aspect of this book and was delightful to work with. Thanks to Sarah Avinger and her team for the layout and cover art. BenBella is a great publisher and I am delighted to be working with them. Many people at BenBella played a part in this book, and I thank you all for your insights, advice, and contributions.

A really special thank-you must go to Silvia Mischler for her invaluable encouragement, creative guidance, and professional direction. You helped bring this project to life and refined it in every step of the process.

A deep, heartfelt thanks to Cherry Wills, CEO and Head Practitioner in Australia and New Zealand, and also the Global Chief Coaching Officer for Metabolic Balance. I so appreciate your leadership to help spread the magic of Metabolic Balance to every corner of the world. Your support of this book is helping to make all the difference. Thanks for your wisdom, patience, and inspiration.

I would like to thank all the Metabolic Balance National License Holders in the world for the work you are doing. Many of you contributed recipes to this book and I thank you for your valuable contributions. I'd also like to thank those at the Metabolic Balance Head Office for allowing me to use the name and logo of this incredible program. And a very special thanks to Rainer H. Keller for your consideration and wonderful support for this project.

When I met Dr. Wolf Funfack on multiple occasions, I found him to be very warm, inspiring, and gracious. His mission was to bring the knowledge of Metabolic Balance to as many doctors and nutritionists as possible, and I am humbled to help share his work with others. I thank him profusely for his influence on my life, and I thank his wife, Birgit Funfack, as well, for her many contributions to Metabolic Balance.

Thanks to Silvia Bürkle, the Metabolic Balance Specialist in Nutrition, for your professional guidance and your continued research to keep Metabolic Balance at the leading edge of nutrition and science. Your support for all the Metabolic Balance coaches around the world is invaluable. Your review of this book is also greatly appreciated and I value your input and wisdom.

Susan Schroeter was the nutritionist who told me about Dr. Wolf Funfack's lecture in Toronto in 2013. And my friend Jeff Michener is the one who insisted that I meet Susan. We may have no idea how important the connections we make in life will ultimately be. Thank you both, so much.

I also want to acknowledge Vera Jamin-Wirth, National License Holder for Metabolic Balance Canada, who helped me establish my Metabolic Balance practice. Thanks to Sylvia Egel for your contributions to this book and continued support in the USA. Dr. Ira Bernstein has also been there for me every step of the way as a medical adviser. Together, they have taught me so many valuable things that continue to influence my success with this awesome program.

Todd Hewitt deserves a huge thanks for encouraging and assisting me with my practice in Hong Kong and for supporting and inspiring me in my expanding practice. Todd, you're a great friend and I thrive in your presence.

Thank you to Mike Day for the beautiful photos, and to LeeAnne Wright, whose food styling was not only incredible to watch, I also truly appreciate the love and care you took with each recipe. You had me in awe. In addition, thanks to Sheila Marcello, who was instrumental in helping with the vision for this book and added her keen insights and support.

I have deep appreciation for the thousands of clients I have worked with over the years. I have learned so much from you and your success and I am so happy you chose me to be a part of your health journey.

To Paul, my husband of over 40 years, I offer my gratitude for your easygoing and supportive assistance every step of the way. When our house was turned upside down as we tested all the recipes for this book, with food, plates, and pots and pans everywhere, you just smiled and cheered me on. To my parents, my three boys, my grandchildren, and my entire huge family and my friends all over the globe, thank you for loving and encouraging me and continually inspiring me to be my best, to want the best, and to always expect the best.

––––––––

The Metabolic Balance license holders in each country and the coaches they work with are available as resources all over the world to help ensure each individual's success with the Metabolic Balance program. If you have questions or want a personalized Metabolic Balance program in your country, please reach out to me at jane@creativehealth.ca and I will assist you or help you find a coach in your area.

In alphabetical order by primary country:

AUSTRALIA/NEW ZEALAND Cherry Wills
BRAZIL Melissa Pancini
BULGARIA Kalina Kirilova
CANADA Vera Jamin-Wirth & Jen Vasey
CROATIA/SERBIA/BOSNIA-HERZEGOVINA/
    MONTENEGRO/SLOVENIA Dr. Nela Roje
CZECH REPUBLIC Ivana Büttner
FRANCE Laurent Causse
GERMANY/AUSTRIA/SWITZERLAND Metabolic
    Balance HQ
HONG KONG Jane Durst-Pulkys
HUNGARY/SLOVAKIA Katarina Grich
INDIA Dr. Gerd Müller & Taranjeet Kaur
IRAN Couros Kamal
ITALY Daniela Langellotti
KENYA/TANZANIA/RWANDA/UGANDA/
    BURUNDI/SOUTH SUDAN Shelina Mediratta
MEXICO Alejandra Merlo
MOROCCO Silvia Mischler
NETHERLANDS Pascale Aschebrock
OMAN/KUWAIT/SAUDI-ARABIA/BAHRAIN/
    QATAR/UAE Artemis Spörri
PERU Deidad Vernal
POLAND Ela Nawrot
PORTUGAL Maria Manuel Frois
ROMANIA /REPUBLICA MOLDOVA Dr. Michaela
    Stein
SOUTH AFRICA Dr. Andreas te Reh
SPAIN Itxaso Mendizabal
TURKEY/AZERBAIJAN Sophie Kamuran Demirtas
UKRAINE Olga & Valentin Tschebrukova
UNITED KINGDOM/IRELAND Gloria Parfitt
USA Sylvia Egel

Testimonials

"Jane Durst-Pulkys has inspired us with her wealth of knowledge and enthusiasm. We found her program easy to follow, and we love the food and recipes. My health issues have been minimized, and I dropped the needed weight! I highly recommend Jane and her new cookbook, *The Metabolic Balance Kitchen*!"
Dr. Victor Abdullah

"At 53 years old, I started experiencing menopause with insomnia, weight gain, skin issues, and hormonal imbalances. I used Jane's program—and I have never seen results like this before! I have been on and off every diet, but this program works! I lost 20 pounds in 4 weeks, my menopause symptoms disappeared, and I gained so much energy . . . I can't wait to try these recipes in Jane's new book! They look fantastic."
Nina Popadic, dental hygienist

"I'm so excited to try the recipes in *The Metabolic Balance Kitchen*! I love that it's full of insights and tips on eating an anti-inflammatory diet and explains exactly how to reset your metabolism. Jane Durst-Pulkys is a great health coach, and I'm sure everyone who reads this book will love it."
Sarah A. Archer, social media consultant

"Jane Durst-Pulkys' new book, *The Metabolic Balance Kitchen*, is powerful. The recipes and information will help people everywhere understand how to reduce inflammation while eating delicious foods! Eliminating excess fat and pain in the body is an advantage almost everyone can appreciate. Jane's positive health advice and incredible energy are reflected in every recipe!"
Henry Koster, owner of Floating Away wellness spa

"Inflammation and weight gain are an epidemic in the United States. Jane's recipes for a healthy and effective Metabolic Balance diet are fabulous. This new cookbook will be a great international success because it contains recipes that will be loved by people everywhere."
Lorry Koster, acupuncturist

"Now everyone can access Jane's exciting recipes for greater health and happiness. We are excited about *The Metabolic Balance Kitchen* and can't wait to share it with others!"
Lynda Kosowan, executive director of Scarborough Women's Centre

"When I first learned about Jane, my life was stressful, and my stomach was always upset; I had psoriasis on both legs, and my hands ached. Jane shared her recipes, added a few supplements, made a few subtle suggestions, and I was on my way to greatly improved health . . . I am so excited to have *The Metabolic Balance Kitchen* as a resource for the great recipes that Jane shares!"
Carol Grellette, retired executive at Dell Computers

"I highly recommend Jane's new cookbook! I had followed a variety of diet programs, and none worked. My condition was aggravated by hypothyroid disease and type 2 diabetes . . . With Jane's recipes, I have been able to maintain my weight easily, and my doctor has eliminated diabetes medicine, reduced cholesterol medicine by half, and even made small adjustments to my thyroid medicine!"
Judith Tse, retired banking executive

"Metabolic Balance changed my life! As a health practitioner myself, I needed some tweaking and a coach to help me reach my health goals . . . This Metabolic Balance cookbook is exactly what I was looking for. Individual recipes that are easy to prepare and totally satisfying. I travel a lot and find it easy to incorporate the program wherever I go."
Barb Burke, holistic health practitioner and herbal therapist

"Jane Durst-Pulkys' cookbook will be a blessing to many! I started the Metabolic Balance program because of chronic pain for years with fibromyalgia. Now, I feel no pain! I am very pleased to have lost 46 pounds, and I feel great!"
Rose Rea, executive at Skyservice

"In 2021, I was at my lowest point and my highest weight ever. Following Jane's advice and her recipes taught me how to eat properly and take care of myself. I lost 38 pounds in 4 months and never felt better. So glad about Jane's new cookbook, *The Metabolic Balance Kitchen*."
Angie Lijoi, administrator

"For anyone who wants to eat healthily and create a routine with measurable results and consistent progress, I highly recommend Jane Durst-Pulkys and her program of Metabolic Balance. Her recipes are fantastic, and her cookbook will be a big winner!"
Joanna Grace, professional musician

"Jane is wise and full of joy, energy, and awareness. All that and more is reflected in this cookbook, *The Metabolic Balance Kitchen*. It is full of sage advice, powerful dietary information, and great tips for improved health!"
Anne Archer, author, editor, and marketing executive

"Following Jane's Metabolic Balance program and the recipes she provides in *The Metabolic Balance Kitchen*, I am healthier, happier, and look ten years younger! My husband and family agree that it was the best thing for me!"
Bonnie Masina, business executive

"I started on Jane's Metabolic Balance program because I was so impressed with her confidence and total conviction. I just had to try it, and I am so glad I did! Jane will help her readers to have a better life from the inside out with this wonderful new cookbook."
Heather Holbrook, graphic artist

"Jane is an excellent coach, mentor, role model, and advisor—and a friend. From every appointment we have had, I have learned something from Jane that positively impacts my life and health. I appreciate all her advice and feel it is perfectly tailored for me and my current goals."
Amber Choudhry, managing director at Debt Capital Markets

"Following the [Metabolic Balance] meal plan that was designed specifically for me, I dropped 30 pounds. I had more energy, and my test results related to health issues had improved dramatically . . . I am very excited to try the many recipes in *The Metabolic Balance Kitchen* and look forward to continued health with this exciting program."
Leo Grellete, chief building official

"*The Metabolic Balance Kitchen* is not only informative, but the recipes are flavorful and easy to make. Metabolic Balance allows me to eat delicious food that lowers inflammation, improves my health, and increases my energy—and helps me achieve my life goals."
Jacqueline Meiers, investment banker

"Jane Durst-Pulkys is an outstanding holistic practitioner. Her overview of health is quite comprehensive, and she's always on the cutting edge. She offers an excellent program for individuals and corporations who want to keep their staff healthy and full of energy and youthful vitality."
Alden Butcher, producer and writer

Index

About the Author

Jane Durst-Pulkys, PhD, is a clinical and holistic nutritionist, author, educator, international speaker, and life coach. She is the Metabolic Balance Brand Ambassador for the United States and specializes in weight management practices in Canada, the USA, and Hong Kong. Her clinical focus includes resetting the metabolism, reducing inflammation, balancing hormones, and achieving optimal weight. She is a nutritional coach for physicians and therapists, works with athletes, advises corporate executives, and consults with people from all walks of life worldwide.

Jane also advises clients as an energy medicine practitioner and believes that health begins with an awareness of one's emotional well-being. Fortune 500 companies find Jane's wellness and health management programs to be extremely valuable for their executives and employees.

Jane is a faculty member and adviser for the Institute of Holistic Nutrition in Toronto and an authority on health and peak performance. With more than 40 years of practical experience, Jane is on the leading edge of proactive approaches to personal health and speaks about health and wellness internationally. She is also the author of *The Book on Confidence* and a frequent guest on television and radio. (www.creativehealth.ca)

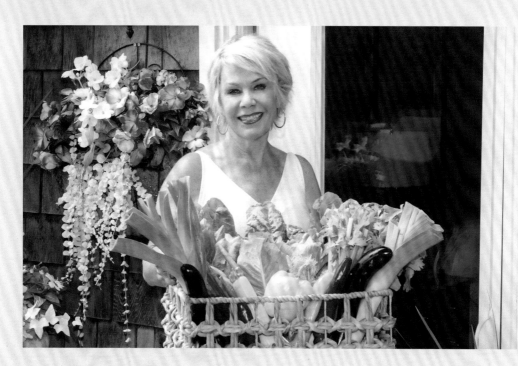